FIONA K

2 weeks

in the ★ ★ ★ ★ ★

FAST LANE

Diet

www.fionakirk.com

NEW 2 WEEKS IN THE FAST LANE DIET
BY FIONA KIRK

NOTE TO READERS

If you are pregnant, breastfeeding, on regular medication, have concerns about your health or are If you are pregnant, breastfeeding, on regular medication, have concerns about your health or are under the age of 16 you should consult your doctor or health practitioner before embarking on any new eating and/or exercise programme. Every effort has been made to present the information in this book in a clear, complete and accurate manner, however not every situation can be anticipated and the information in this book cannot take the place of a medical analysis of individual health needs. The author and Painless Publishing hereby disclaim any and all liability resulting from injuries or damage caused by following any recommendations in this book.

REFERENCES

All statements (other than personal views) and studies referred to throughout the book have been exhaustively researched but the author chose not to reference them throughout the text and add copious additional pages at the back of the book. Should you wish further information about any of the above, email through the author's website *fionakirk.com* and they will be provided promptly.

CONTRIBUTORS

Design and Typesetting: Max Morris, Milkbar Creative *milkbar-creative.com*
eBook Creation: Alan Cooper *yourebookpartners.com*

Contents

CHANGING
THE WAY
we Shift Fat
forever

Introduction

I devised the **2 Weeks in the Fast Lane** diet in 2010 as part of my very first book, **So What the F*** Should I Eat?** and such was the enthusiasm for this quick fix (and healthy) diet that I was goaded into publishing it independently in 2011. It has proved extremely popular and I have received countless emails from dieters from all corners of the globe enthusing about the diet and regaling me with interesting stories about how they have not only achieved their weight/fat loss goal but maintained it by sticking with some or all of my recommendations which is music to my ears!

So Why Update it?

Surely if it isn't broken, it doesn't need fixing? Well... largely as a result of the so-called *obesity crisis* worldwide and the extremely worrying health threats posed by being overweight or clinically obese, research into diet, eating and lifestyle habits has gone into orbit with increasing funds being dedicated to finding out where it has all gone so horribly wrong and what we should do in a bid to reverse the unfolding drama.

It is a veritable minefield and hard to stay abreast of but I have always promised my readers and followers that through my website, my blog, my newsletters and via social media, I will keep them up to date with research - some of which is extremely reliable, some of which is emerging but still needs further investigation and some of which is downright irresponsible and should never make it out of the lab, never mind onto the front pages of the press which does little other than instil an element of panic and create further confusion.

So... what better time than now to bring the **2 Weeks in the Fast Lane** diet right up to speed with a wealth of research-backed changes we can all make over the space of two weeks to make fat loss a reality rather than a vague hope!

Food For Thought

Anyone who is familiar with my 'writings' on the subject of diets and fat loss will be familiar with the phrase 'little changes reap big rewards' as I invariably advocate you do just that - make a few gradual changes and once you get comfortable with them and they start to become habit, make a few more.

However, whilst I still believe this is a surefire route to successful fat loss, I have become increasingly alert to the fact that the combination of changes is vitally important which is why this new updated *2 Weeks in the Fast Lane* diet not only concentrates on change but also encourages you to make as many changes as you can in just two weeks to really get the ball rolling.

Consider this: it's all well and good if you get into the habit of snacking on yoghurt and fruit or light broths instead of salty snacks and fizzy drinks or lattes and pastries but you are likely to come a cropper if you continue to have sugary cereals for breakfast most mornings or pasta for dinner four nights a week or only exercise once a week.

It is the combination of the changes that make the real difference

In a Nutshell!

Here is what I am proposing:

Make 10 Changes Starting Today

Make 6 Changes Within 2 Weeks

Make 4 Changes As You Move Forward

Some are relatively straightforward and shouldn't cause much angst, others may be a little harder - but - if you don't nail them all, don't fret, just have a go and keep having a go!

The somewhat pessimistic French quote *plus ça change, plus c'est la même chose* (the more things change, the more they stay the same) has absolutely no place when it comes to diet and health. It is crystal clear to me that diets have to change if we want to live a long and healthy life and by that I mean a life that doesn't involve us becoming disabled with one of the many degenerative diseases for the last 5, 10, 15 or even 20 years of our life.

I am crucially aware that many of us lead very busy lives and with that in mind, I rarely (if ever) recommend diets that involve vast numbers of foods and beverages that are difficult to source, expensive to buy or which you have to force down - I leave that to others!

However, you will come across the odd morsel that you may be unfamiliar with but I urge you to try as there is good reason for its inclusion. It may be that it is respected for its fat burning properties or it may be that it is super-rich in health-enhancing and/or health-protective nutrients or it may simply be that I believe it adds something extra special to one of the many recipes I spend copious hours experimenting with to provide you with delicious, nutritious and satisfying plates of food!

Just promise me you will make a huge effort to embrace change!

Are you in the habit of believing that 'going on a diet' where fat loss is the goal means deprivation, hunger, sugar cravings, boring repetition of dull and unexciting foods and the removal of everything you love?

HOLD THAT THOUGHT!

That's never going to work for much more than a week or two before you throw in the towel. No diet is ever going to work long term if you don't look forward to daily meals and snacks, really enjoy the 'eating experience' and feel energised and satisfied after each and every one you take a little care and a lot of love over shopping for, preparing, cooking and/or selecting when you are out and about!

Allow me to 'take the dismal out of dieting' by offering you a wealth of tried, tested and in many cases, proven changes you can make to your diet which can make a monumental difference and encourage daily fat loss.

IT'S EASIER THAN YOU MIGHT THINK!

Let's Start with a Quiz?

Who doesn't like a quiz? But let me be clear here. It's not a test, no-one is going to 'pull you up' if you get a few answers incorrect or simply don't understand the question - and - it's certainly not designed to result in you feeling in any way inadequate because your nutritional knowledge is perhaps a little scant!

No... the aim here is to allow you to ascertain the areas pertaining to your diet where there is more than a little confusion! Let me reiterate. Finding a diet (in the true sense of the word - ie. a 'way of life') that suits you, suits your timetable, suits your lifestyle, suits your tastes, prompts fat loss until you reach your 'happy' weight and enables you to maintain it requires real focus and determination for a spell before it can become second nature.

IMPORTANT!

My goal is to arm you with the knowledge that is going to allow you to change a number of practices that play a major role in improving your health and wellbeing and remind your body that there's work to be done!

We are pre-wired to store fat to ensure we have sufficient energy to get us through the 'lean times' which our early ancestors had to deal with on a regular basis to keep them alive but sadly, it hasn't moved on, hasn't gotten to grips with the fact that many of us are now lucky enough to live in 'the land of plenty' where food is all around us and 'lean times' are unlikely, so it just keeps on squirrelling it away! The message you need to shout loud and clear to your often-confused body when you want to lose weight is "don't panic, it's all good, I'm providing you with an excellent balance of nourishment at least 3 times a day so it's ok to release some of that stored fat to stoke the metabolic fire!"

How Much Do You Know?

If you get 12 or more answers correct you are clearly well up to speed! (answers at the back of the book)

1. **Which early morning meal will best keep hunger at bay until lunchtime?**
   a) a fruit and yoghurt smoothie
   b) a bowl of Cheerios with milk
   c) scrambled eggs on rye toast
   d) a breakfast cereal bar
   e) toast and marmalade/jam

2. A portion of which of the following offers the highest levels of immune-boosting vitamin C?

   a) bananas
   b) berries
   c) broccoli
   d) oranges

3. Which type of milk is most commonly associated with lactose intolerance and digestive complaints?

   a) almond milk
   b) cows milk
   c) goats milk
   d) coconut milk

4. Which of the following snacks is most likely to create a 'sugar rush'?

   a) a bunch of grapes and a few slices of cheese
   b) an energy bar and a can of diet cola
   c) an iced doughnut and a cup of tea
   d) a pack of mixed nuts, seeds and dried fruit

5. Which of the following is our richest food source of health-enhancing vitamin D?

   a) beans
   b) cabbage
   c) oily fish
   d) avocado

6. Which of the following offers the greatest levels of Omega 3 fats per 100g?

   a) spinach
   b) walnuts
   c) sunflower seeds

7. Which vitamin is associated with good eye health?

    a) vitamin B2
    b) vitamin A
    c) vitamin K
    d) vitamin E

8. Which animal meat has the least saturated fat per 100g?

    a) beef
    b) lamb
    c) chicken
    d) venison

9. Which spice has shown itself to give the body the biggest metabolic boost when included in meals and snacks?

    a) ginger
    b) cinnamon
    c) mustard
    d) chilli
    e) nutmeg

10. Which of the following plant foods is richest in health-enhancing 'resistant' starch?

    a) bok choy
    b) beans
    c) squash
    d) peppers

11. Which of the following is an excellent source of the blood sugar balancing mineral chromium?

    a) green beans
    b) oats
    c) broccoli

12. Which of these foods provides a 'complete' protein (ie. contains all the essential amino acids)?

a) adzuki beans
b) puy lentils
c) chia seeds
d) chickpeas

13. Which of the following drinks (per glass) has the least number of calories?

a) coconut water
b) hot chocolate
c) cola
d) orange juice

14. In addition to calcium, which other mineral is vital to good bone health?

a) zinc
b) magnesium
c) potassium

15. Which of the following meals offers the healthiest balance of protein, fats and carbohydrates?

a) baked potato stuffed with bacon and cheese
b) poached egg on a base of mushroom, spinach, avocado and smoked salmon
c) spaghetti with tomato and herb sauce
d) chicken curry with white basmati rice

16. Which of the following belongs to the group known as 'nightshade vegetables'?

a) carrots
b) beetroot
c) peppers
d) cabbage

17. How many hours of sleep per night are linked to deteriorating health and weight gain over time?

    a) 5 to 6
    b) 7 to 8
    c) 8 to 9

18. Which of the following lunches are most likely to make you feel drowsy in the afternoon?

    a) fish soup
    b) pizza margherita
    c) quinoa and vegetable salad
    d) baked potato with chilli and sour cream

19. For strong and healthy hair and nails we need good levels of zinc in our diet. Which of the following is a rich source of this mineral?

    a) sweet potato
    b) olives
    c) mushrooms
    d) aubergine

20. Which of the following is our richest source of heart-friendly monounsaturated fats?

    a) eggs
    b) olives
    c) walnuts
    d) oily fish

What Have You Tried So Far?

LET'S TALK DIETS!

Which weight loss diets have you had a go at? The Fast diet, the Paleo diet, the Mediterranean diet, some sort of Sugar-Free or Gluten-Free diet, an Alkaline diet, the DASH diet, the Weight Watchers diet, the SIRT diet or any one of the many fad diets involving all manner of slightly unusual eating practices and equally many guaranteed weight loss promises that dominate the media for a time with case studies showing willing victims who have 'allegedly' lost anywhere between 2 and 5 stones in just a matter of months and have never looked back!

Did any of them work? Are you now that person who is in that enviable place where "the diet starts Monday" is no longer a statement you utter either to yourself or to others? I have a sneaking suspicion that the answer is no, otherwise I doubt you would be reading this book! Having said that, I imagine there are at least a few of the diets you have tried which 'delivered the goods' (ie. weight loss was achieved in the short term but not in the long term) and ultimately it was back to square one before the desperate search began again for another route which was going to make permanent fat loss really happen.

GOOD NEWS! THERE ARE WAYS TO GET OUT OF THE DIET TRAP?

I have no issue with quick fix diets - many work well and research now indicates that when we see impressive weight loss in the first week or so, we are much more likely to stick with the plan for longer - and - as we feel better, look leaner and have more energy, we are more likely to continue to factor many of the diet recommendations into our lives on a daily basis. But (and this is a very big but), if any diet we launch into is in any way short of the kind of nourishment the body needs to ensure that its health is not compromised, it can become a mighty struggle to 'stick to the rules'. We become tired, we become fractious, we can't concentrate, our sleep is disrupted, we fall prey to every bug or virus that is 'doing the rounds' and perhaps worst of all, we become horribly-bored with the diet!

WHEN DID YOU LAST TURN THINGS UPSIDE DOWN OR RIGHT AROUND?

Some say us humans don't much like change but I would challenge that! We regularly have to adapt to change throughout our lives. We change little things like adopting a new hairstyle or having a go with the latest clothing fashions or simply rearranging the furniture in the front room and we change bigger things like moving house, going for jobs that are possibly out of our comfort zone, emigrating to another country or getting out of difficult relationships and whilst some work out and others don't, generally-speaking we can give ourselves at least a small pat on the back because we 'gave it a go'. But we don't seem to be quite so good at changing our eating habits!

IS FOOD THE CONSTANT, THE RELIABLE AND THE ONE BIG DEPENDABLE?

No matter how bad things are, there is always the promise of a bit of comfort in the form of a Friday night takeaway or a tub of Ben and Jerrys at the movies or the stress-relieving bag of salty, crunchy and moreish Kettle crisps with a glass of beer or wine at the end of a crazy day or a steaming hot and syrupy caramel latte on a cold morning. When the chips are down, the mac and cheese beats the lentil and bean salad every time and when the diet isn't going well, it's usually the sticky pastry rather than the piece of fruit that beckons!

HAVE YOU HEARD OF THE BLUE ZONES?

These are the parts of the world where people have either lived or are likely to live past their 100th birthday. As researcher and writer Dan Buettner writes in his book **The Blue Zones**, *"The world's longevity all-stars not only live longer, they also tend to live better. They have strong connections with their family and friends. They are active. They wake up in the morning knowing that they have a purpose and the world, in turn, reacts to them in a way that propels them along. An overwhelming majority of them still enjoy life."*

Foods that are especially prominent in the diets of the blue zones include vegetables, fruits, herbs, nuts and seeds, beans and legumes, quality fats like olive oil, high-quality dairy products like grass-fed goat milk and homemade cheeses, fermented products like yoghurt, kefir, tempeh, miso and natto, whole grains such as durum wheat or locally grown (organic) corn. Meat is typically eaten only a few times a month while sheep or goats milk, eggs and fish are consumed more often, usually a few times per week. They usually eat animal-based meals on special occasions, such as holidays, festivals or when they have access to meat from neighbourhood farms.

There is so much we can learn from these 'longevity all-stars' but whilst it's all good in theory, it's slightly harder in practice when we live in densely populated areas, work long hours in temperature-controlled offices in large cities, spend copious hours per week in cars or on public transport and have scant time to get food on the table on a daily basis or enjoy outdoor pursuits.

However, with a bit of determination, we can factor at least some of their principles into our lives and now is the time to start!

WHO DOESN'T LOVE AN IMAGE TO WORK WITH WHEN PREPARING A DISH?

Sadly, it is not possible for me to include images of the recipes that I have worked long and hard on and are featured in your diet in this book format but you can find them all on my website **www.fionakirk.com** to hopefully whet your appetite and encourage you to get into the kitchen and 'have a go'! Just click on '**Books**' then '**2 Weeks in the Fast Lane**' then '**Recipe Image Gallery**' and they are all there!

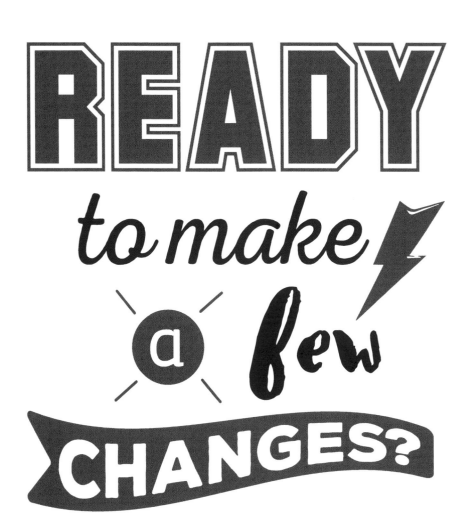

READY to make a few CHANGES?

2

10 Changes to Make Starting Today

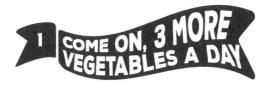

1 COME ON, 3 MORE VEGETABLES A DAY

This advice generally elicits a groan from many who immediately assume this means endless hours of peeling, chopping and steaming followed by endless hours of crunching and chewing their way through platefuls of raw and cooked vegetables but it doesn't have to be that way. There are loads of ways to get 7 portions (my recommendation) into a day by including vegetables not just as a 'side' to other foods but also in soups, stews, salads, sauces and juices.

HERE'S A SAMPLE DAY TO PROVE IT....

BREAKFAST
a lettuce, spinach, cucumber, pear and melon smoothie alongside your scrambled egg on toast

MID MORNING
a selection of raw baby vegetables with a small pot of red pepper hummus

LUNCH
a chicken and vegetable broth with a greek salad

MID AFTERNOON
half an avocado stuffed with tuna or cottage cheese

DINNER
fish, parcel-baked with spinach, onions, and tomatoes with stir fried thai-style greens alongside

That's in excess of 7 portions and not only does it constitute a delicious day's eating but indicates just how easy it is to include vegetables in many different ways.

WHY ARE VEGETABLES SO IMPORTANT?

- they are so low in calories that it is difficult to gain weight even if you overeat them

- they are an exceptionally rich source of water-soluble vitamins and since the body cannot make these and we need a good daily supply, we have to get them from the food we eat

- they offer an abundance of phytonutrients, the plant chemicals that give foods their brilliant colours, their delicious flavours and their unique aromas. These are the nutrients most closely linked to prevention of many diseases

- they are some of the richest sources of fibre available in the plant kingdom. Fibre-rich foods promote healthy digestion and elimination

- they are rich in anti-inflammatory compounds. Inflammation is at the root of most diseases that plague our society and the evidence is clear that anti-inflammatory foods can regulate the immune system and have a positive impact on the way inflammation affects our bodies

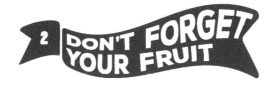

2 DON'T FORGET YOUR FRUIT

Fruit has taken a bit of bashing recently which is not only shocking but also short-sighted. Some suggest we should seriously reduce our fruit consumption and this is largely because fruit is rich in fructose and too much fructose in our diet has been linked to an increasing number of health issues and weight gain over time. But, fresh fruit isn't just about fructose, it is also a great source of fibre and water and is rich in protective plant chemicals, some of which we don't get from other foods so to simply lump them into the same category as the vast array of fructose-heavy processed foods that line the shelves is overly-simplistic to say the least.

I say get 2 or 3 portions into your day, remember that the skin and seeds are where the protective plant chemicals are concentrated so don't peel them unless you have to and in a bid to ensure that their sugars don't play havoc with your blood sugar, always have some protein/fat alongside (nuts, seeds, cheese, meat, poultry, yoghurt etc) and enjoy every sweet and syrupy bite!

You will find a goodly selection of meal and snack suggestions in your diet plan that include fruit and as long as you stick to the recommendations and have no more than 2 or 3 portions per day, the benefits vastly outweigh any concerns about consuming too much fructose.

Fresh fruit juices are the ones to watch however (and should be counted as part of your daily portions) but if you stick to the following guidelines, all will be well:

- juice your own or always ensure that 'off the shelf' varieties are as natural as possible with no added sugars
- always water fresh fruit juices down 50:50 with still or sparkling water
- always have a little protein or fat alongside

Please Note...

Those of you who have read and followed the original 2 Weeks in the Fast Lane diet which recommended fruit on its own every day until mid morning may be wondering why I am now 'changing the goalposts' a little!

As mentioned in the introduction, things are moving at pace on the nutritional research front and it is now becoming clear that some who struggle to lose weight and/or find it difficult to maintain their initial weight loss often suffer from difficult-to-manage blood sugar peaks and troughs at certain times of the day which may exacerbate sugar cravings. So, in a bid to ensure that you benefit from the important health-enhancing properties of eating fruit on a daily basis whilst avoiding possible blood sugar issues, I believe the best route is to 'play it safe', so I propose the addition of a little protein and/or fat when consuming fruit to slow the delivery of fruit sugars into the bloodstream.

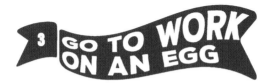

There is scant evidence to prove that skipping breakfast results in us eating more during the remainder of the day and compromising weight loss. It is simply one of the many diet dilemmas that continues to be flagged up! Some of us can't focus or get on with our day without breakfast, others function just fine until they are actually hungry which may well be an hour or two into our day.

The first thing you should be alert to is that for many of us, breakfasting is a habit - we have been doing it for so long that we rarely question it and simply scarf something down at pace before we go out the door. Only you can determine whether you actually need it or not and if you do, you must ensure that it counts.

The most common mistake people make is to eat typical breakfast foods, many of which are highly processed and loaded with sugars - cereals, toast, waffles, muffins, bagels etc which satisfy hunger for a short time but not for long and before you know it, an energy dip occurs and you start thinking about a snack.

Another mistake those who have become aware of the damaging effect of excess starchy carbohydrates and sugar make, is overdosing on protein but ignoring fats. A protein-rich breakfast is certainly going to keep blood sugar levels balanced for longer than a starch-rich breakfast and help to avoid hunger and cravings mid to late morning but if you are really serious about losing weight and prompting day-long fat burning, do yourself a favour and get some fats in there! No, they are not fattening, no, they don't prompt unhealthy cholesterol levels and no, they don't increase your risk of heart disease.

What they do, when eaten regularly but in small but meaningful amounts is fill you up, help to satisfy your appetite, please the palate and boost the action of the enzymes that encourage fat burning.

You will note in your diet plan that rather than pinpointing 'breakfast', I am calling it your 'first meal of the day'. For some, this may indeed be somewhere within the first hour of getting up, for others it may well be an hour or so later. Only you can decide when you start to feel hungry. It often depends on what you had for dinner the previous evening - some days you wake up needing sustenance, other days you don't so don't be a slave to the breakfast habit.

So why do I champion eggs for your first meal of the day (or indeed, any time of the day)?

- Eggs are a 'complete' protein - ie. they contain all the essential amino acids (the building blocks of a protein). Two whole eggs offer around 12 grams of protein

- Two whole eggs offer around 10 grams of health-enhancing and filling fat

- They are rich in energy-generating B vitamins, particularly choline which is used to build cell membranes and plays an important role in producing signalling molecules in the brain

- Egg yolks contain good levels of the powerful antioxidants, lutein and zeaxanthin which build up in the retina of the eye. Studies show that consuming adequate amounts of these nutrients can significantly reduce the risk of cataracts and macular degeneration

- Eggs score high on a scale called the 'satiety index' which measures the ability of foods to induce feelings of fullness and reduce subsequent calorie intake. In one study of 30 overweight women, eating eggs instead of bagels for breakfast increased feelings of fullness and resulted in them eating fewer calories for the next 36 hours and in another study, replacing a bagel with an egg for breakfast caused significant weight loss over a period of 8 weeks

You will find an excellent selection of egg dishes for meal and snack choices within your diet plan and in the recipe section. But for those of you who don't eat eggs, there are plenty of protein and fat-rich morning alternatives.

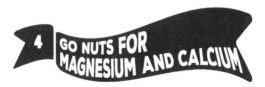

4 GO NUTS FOR MAGNESIUM AND CALCIUM

Probably the best known 'courting couple' in the mineral world and vital for strong bones and teeth, muscle function, a healthy heart, a sharp brain, nerve transmission, restful sleep, good digestion and elimination and valuable weight loss or weight management. But, Western diets all too often provide the body with rather too much calcium and not enough magnesium which can upset the delicate balance between the two and prompt health issues.

Enter the humble nut! Not only do nuts provide good levels of these important minerals, but also offer them in good ratios (ie. impressive levels of magnesium and respectable but not over-zealous levels of calcium).

Many fear nuts, believing them to be 'fattening' and yes, if you don't watch your daily portions, you may compromise weight loss - but - a couple of handfuls per day as snacks or toppings or in the form of sugar-free nut butters can make a forcible difference.

Epidemiological studies show that nut consumers tend to be leaner than those who do not regularly consume nuts and furthermore, suggest that nuts can be incorporated into the diet without the risk of weight gain (and in some cases, induce weight loss) and more importantly, greatly improve diet quality. The rationale to date is as follows:

- Nuts are high in protein and fibre with a low glycaemic index value, which may promote satiety resulting in a reduction in calories consumed from other foods.

- The crunchy textural property of whole nuts may also promote satiety as the mechanical act of mastication results in the secretion of appetite-suppressing hormones.

- Nut consumption may lead to an increase in energy expenditure - the high unsaturated fat content of nuts may increase our resting metabolic rate (RMR).

- Some of the fat found in nuts may not be highly bio-accessible meaning that a high proportion of this fat is excreted in the faeces.

AND DON'T FORGET SEEDS!

Seeds of all types also offer an excellent ratio of magnesium to calcium as do greens, spinach, bok choy, chard, kale, cabbage, broccoli, Brussels sprouts, blackstrap molasses and beans so if you have an allergy or intolerance, there's still plenty to choose from. Nuts, seeds and all of the above plus a few extras are regularly included in your diet plan to ensure you get plenty of both, carefully balanced.

MAGNESIUM AND WEIGHT LOSS

Magnesium assists in keeping body fluids balanced, thereby reducing the chance of water retention, plays an important role in managing the level of sugar in our bloodstream, thereby reducing the invasion of energy dips and food cravings and it also helps to relax muscles in the digestive tract, thereby enhancing the absorption of nutrients into the bloodstream and reducing the likelihood of constipation.

TOP MAGNESIUM-RICH FOODS:

Greens - the greener the better!

Beans - all types

Nuts - a little goes a long way!

Seeds - make it daily!

Tofu - a great meat alternative!

Quinoa - top grain for protein!

Oats - a spectacular grain!

Ancient grains - experiment!

Berries - the brightest and the best!

CALCIUM AND WEIGHT LOSS

A growing body of evidence indicates that a diet rich in calcium allows us to burn more calories per day. There is also some evidence that when calcium levels in the body are low the brain detects this and stimulates feelings of hunger, causing us to eat more. Conversely, medium to high levels transmit signals to the brain indicating that we are full, suppressing the desire to eat more.

Diets that include medium to high levels of calcium-rich foods have been found to result in up to half the amount of fat being stored to those providing low levels. This is believed to be as a direct result of calcium having the ability to reduce the action of a life-preserving enzyme system within the body which encourages fat storage.

It has also been suggested that increased calcium in the diet may reduce the transport of fat from the intestines into the bloodstream. The calcium binds with bile acids and increases the transport of fat from the intestines into the bloodstream. This action also increases the amount of fat we excrete through the bowel so instead of storing it we lose it!

LOW = less than 600mg per day

MEDIUM = 600-1000mg per day

HIGH = 1000mg plus per day

TOP CALCIUM-RICH FOODS:

Spinach - bursting with calcium and magnesium!

Tofu - it's all about the soya beans!

Natural Yoghurt - make it a daily habit!

Sesame seeds and Tahini

Cheese - great for a small snack!

Tinned and fresh Sardines

Greens - the more the better!

Cinnamon - great sprinkled over porridge!

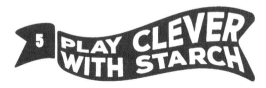

I'm afraid the news is not good if you are planning on shedding those excess pounds of fat and are one of those types who tend to like your food (no matter how fresh and colourful and health-enhancing it may be!) wrapped up in a flat bread, packed between two slices of bread or toast or a bagel or a buttery croissant, accompanied by a mound of pasta, noodles or rice, served on a bed of creamy potato mash, enveloped in pastry or fried in batter!

Many of the above that many eat on a regular basis involve refined flour and refined flour products have a very similar effect on the body to sugar. Because most of the nutrients and fibre have been lost during the refining process, we are left with little other than chains of sugar (glucose) which don't hang around in the stomach too long, are pretty quickly 'unchained' in the small intestine, are released into the bloodstream then ferried off to body cells to generate energy. Hence the reason, a bowl of cornflakes or a slice of toast before you rush out the door in the morning stems your hunger for a while - but not for long! Because the whole process happens in a flash (courtesy of the fact that there is not much other than rapidly-digested sugars for the body to get to work on), it's more than likely that hunger and possibly an invasive sugar craving will enter the stage by mid morning (same applies to mid afternoon if you have grabbed a sandwich or wrap or bagel for lunch) and this is absolutely not what you need or want when you are trying to lose weight!

There is now universal agreement that keeping a healthy balance of glucose in the bloodstream throughout the day and night is the way to go for a healthy body, a healthy weight and a sharp brain.

So, the big question is: do you actually need starchy carbohydrates in your daily diet? The very low carb advocates say "no - you can get all the essentials the body needs from protein, fats, plants and water" but this kind of diet requires a deal of dedication to ensure that we get our full quota of energy-generating nutrients and digestion-enhancing fibre into our day so my advice is to include those that are as natural and unrefined as possible but don't let them play a major role in any meal or snack.

Here are the carbohydrate foods you should concentrate on and why:

- Greens and cruciferous vegetables are particularly noted for helping protect the body from many cancers.

- Brightly coloured vegetables and fruits are rich in plant chemicals which counteract free radical damage and help to naturally slow ageing.

- The richness of fibre in root vegetables slows the release of glucose, controls appetite and delays hunger.

- Sprouted grains, beans and legumes are a powerhouse of energy-stabilising nutrients.

- Sprouted grain breads are deliciously-nourishing, hormone-balancing and easily digested.

- Fruit is a great source of fibre and water and is rich in protective plant chemicals, some of which we don't get from other foods.

- Beans, lentils and legumes are rich in resistant starch which has a low impact on blood sugar and discourages insulin sensitivity.

- Ancient grains are rich in fibre, protein, vitamins, minerals and protective antioxidants and many are gluten-free.

- Nuts and seeds offer an excellent combination of carbohydrate, protein, fat and protective plant chemicals.

You will note that vegetables take the number one spot for all the reasons previously mentioned, fruit is important, beans, lentils and legumes shouldn't be forgotten, nor should nuts and seeds and whilst starchy grains are included, only those which are going to add substantial nourishment and discourage blood sugar swings are flagged up.

Your diet plan has been carefully designed in such a way that you reap the daily benefits of including starches but they don't feature regularly - they only feature in small amounts and those that are included are your best bet nutritionally.

For those of you who exercise regularly and strenuously in the evening before your evening meal, there are also recommendations in your diet plan on which unrefined starches to include to safeguard muscle glycogen levels and counteract the all-consuming hunger that often invades post-exercise and prompts us to wolf down a huge plate of pasta!

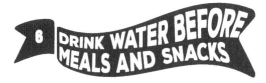

There are a couple of very good reasons for this. Firstly, it makes perfect sense biochemically. Nearly every chemical reaction that takes place in the body 24/7 requires an aqueous environment. Insufficient water equals a less than impressive chemical reaction and on occasion, no reaction at all. We need water to digest food, carry waste products out of the body, send electrical messages between cells, regulate body temperature, lubricate our moving parts and keep our brain sharp. It's a sobering thought but never forget that we can live without food for weeks but without water we will die in a matter of days so this fact in itself should be sufficient reason for us all to pay attention to our daily fluid intake!

Secondly, getting into the habit of drinking a good glassful of water before we eat helps to ensure we stay well-hydrated throughout the day without having to remember to down a small glass every few hours which can sometimes result in us having to force down a small ponds-worth later in the day when we realise we haven't consumed enough! Plus, research indicates that drinking water before we eat means there is a good chance we will eat less food at one sitting.

There is scant proven research behind this strategy but it works well for many dieters and the way I see it, my job here is to arm you with as many strategies as I can to give you the best possible chance of making every day a fat loss day and for many, this means making sure that gnawing hunger and invasive cravings don't mess with the food choices we make. Another bonus is that while we are drinking that glass of water before we eat, we gain a little extra time to think through just what and how much we really need to eat at each meal or snack to keep us energised and firing on all cylinders until the next time we have to make choices all over again!

IT WORKS FOR MANY AND IT CAN WORK FOR YOU!

You will find recommendations in your diet plan on not only how to make drinking water a little less of a 'daily chore' but also a wealth of other drink suggestions to enjoy on a regular basis.

It is also important to remember that many foods are 'water-rich' and do a sterling job of adding to your daily fluid intake. Here are your top fruits and vegetables, all of which are included in your diet plan:

cucumber	radishes	courgettes
strawberries	salad greens	peppers
grapefruit	watermelon	celery

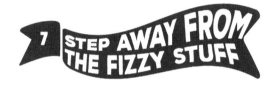

There are just two types of fizzy (carbonated) drinks that get my vote. Sparkling water and *Brut Nature* or *Extra Brut* champagne, prosecco or cava! In my view, all the rest (and this includes all those diet and zero and sugar-free concoctions) should be loaded into a very large space capsule and sent into outer space, never to return.

One of the biggest favours you can do yourself if you want to lose weight and feel and look better in the shortest possible time is to get all but my two recommendations out of your life, starting today!

The full sugar versions of the majority of the fizzy soft drinks and 'sports' drinks that fill the shelves are full of *added* sugars - and the 'diet' versions are full of *artificial* sugars and neither offer any benefit to our health whatsoever.

There has recently been a spate of 'news' suggesting, on the back of a couple of research studies, that no or low calorie colas and the like are better than water when it comes to weight loss - I wonder who funded or part-funded those studies? I think we can all make an educated guess on that one!

To my mind, this is possibly one of the most irresponsible pieces of diet 'news' to hit the headlines for some time. I imagine the goal was to encourage those who regularly drink the **full sugar varieties** to switch to the **diet varieties** and in doing so, consume less sugar but if the aim is to educate us about what we should be eating and drinking to achieve optimum health and where necessary, weight loss, and give us the tools to advise our children on what constitutes a healthy and balanced diet, they should be extremely ashamed of themselves.

And whilst I am having a rant, what could possibly be right about public health authorities advising us to **"swap sugary soft drinks for diet, sugar-free or no added sugar varieties to reduce your sugar intake in a simple step"**? The only thing this kind of advice is going to do is boost the sales of 'diet' drinks and further threaten our health and our waistlines - it's just plain wrong on so very many levels!

What I promised you in the introduction is fat loss and that means **little or no added sugars** and definitely **no artificial sugars** so if you are in the habit of quaffing a couple of cans or bottles in a day and clinging on to the possibility that because 'no added sugars' features in large letters on the label it's all good, sorry but I have to disappoint.

Current findings indicate that whilst *all sugars* trigger enhanced activity within the brain's pleasure centres (and that includes naturally-occurring sugars in whole, unprocessed foods), *artificial sugars* provide less satisfaction so we tend to crave more of them and more sugar in general. This can contribute to not only overeating and weight gain, but also to an unhealthy dependence on sweet and sugary foods and a greater risk of diabetes, heart conditions, strokes and mental decline.

You may already be 'sugar-dependent' and I am not for one minute going to suggest that getting added and/or artificial sugars out of your life is easy but making a determined effort to *step away from the fizzy stuff* is an excellent place to start and can make a huge difference in a short time.

Same goes for a great many non-fizzy soft and sports drinks which are regularly marketed as 'healthy' or 'energy-giving' and some even try to get away with suggesting that they slot into the 'health food' category because they are fortified with vitamins and minerals - not so fast - they are still packed with sugars and there are a lot better ways to get the essential vitamins and minerals into our diet!

First thing to do is always look at labels. Added sugars have a variety of names other than just plain old sugar. Everything that ends in -ose or -ol is sugar as are all syrups and caramels and when it comes to 'diet' drinks, aspartame, cyclamate, saccharin, acesulfame potassium or sucralose are the main artificial sugars involved and then there are usually added artificial colours and flavours - who could possibly get excited about those other than the shareholders of soft drink companies who are raking in the cash on the back of our massive, global, daily consumption?

If you are looking for a few refreshing bubbles, sparkling water should be your go-to and it's extremely easy to brighten it up. You can simply add ice cubes and slices of fresh fruit, vegetables and herbs or you can make one of your favourite smoothies or juices and flask them and when a bit of fizz is called for, go half and half or 60:40 sparkling water and smoothie or juice. Another excellent combination is chilled tea (black, red, green, white, chai, fruit, herb) topped up with sparkling water and perhaps with a drizzle of honey for a little sweetness.

And why do champagne, prosecco and cava feature here? Because the *Brut Nature* and *Extra Brut* varieties are extremely light on sugar (generally a quarter of a teaspoon or less per glass) and if you are aiming for successful fat loss and alcohol is perhaps playing an occasional role in your diet (occasional being the watchword), they are a splendid little treat! Read on for more advice on where alcohol sits on the fat loss front plus a few tips for those who are partial to the odd tipple!

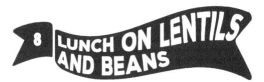

8 LUNCH ON LENTILS AND BEANS

As previously mentioned, a great many starchy foods are rapidly digested and absorbed into the bloodstream. These cause blood glucose levels to rise quickly and drive up the release of insulin, the hormone which is rather too keen on telling the body to make and store fat which is why they should be carefully-controlled if you want to shed fat! These are generally foods made with refined white flour (bread, rolls, cakes, pastries, biscuits, many breakfast cereals).

Then there are the minimally refined/processed starchy foods which take a little longer to be digested and absorbed into the bloodstream but still, if eaten regularly and allowed to play a rather too major role in meals and snacks, also cause blood glucose levels to rise relatively quickly and drive up the release of insulin so also have to be watched when fat loss is the goal. This bunch of starches include brown and wild rice, whole grain pastas and breads, quinoa and 'ancient' grains like teff, amaranth, spelt, faro, millet, kamut, freekeh etc.

FOR SUCCESSFUL FAT LOSS, YOU HAVE TO KNOW YOUR STARCHES!

There is one type of starch that has little effect on blood glucose levels and doesn't drive up the production of insulin which means the body is not encouraged to make and store fat and that is resistant starch. It has rather a lot of names, some call it non-digestible starch, others call it fermentable starch but resistant starch probably best describes its rather splendid properties and I urge you to get to grips with why and how it is important in a health-enhancing and fat busting diet.

It is largely resistant to the digestive process of being broken down into glucose molecules and absorbed through the gut wall into the bloodstream and just carries on down to the colon where it goes through a fermentation process that produces short chain fatty acids (SCAs) which have a number of health benefits:

- They are protective of colon cells and associated with less genetic damage which can lead to cancer.
- They increase mineral absorption, particularly calcium and magnesium which are important for heart and bone health.
- By feeding the healthy bacteria, growth of unhealthy bacteria and their toxic by-products is suppressed.

AND WHEN IT COMES TO FAT LOSS...

- It helps to slow down the pace at which digestible carbohydrates get broken down thereby reducing the counter-productive blood sugar highs and lows which see us reaching for more food.
- It increases satiety, keeping us feeling fuller for longer so we eat less in the course of a day.
- It increases the absorption of magnesium which is linked to reducing fat storage.

- It promotes bowel regularity - constipation is no friend where fat loss is desired.

- It encourages a fabulous phenomenon known as *second meal effect* where the insulin response is controlled not just after a meal rich in resistant starch but also for hours thereafter and well into our next meal resulting in us eating less.

Whilst there are quite a number of foods rich in resistant starch, those that offer the greatest levels and are easiest to fit into a straightforward and easy-to-manage diet are legumes - beans, lentils, split peas and chickpeas so these are what I aim to concentrate on and include in your diet plan.

NB: If you are 'new to legumes', you may find they cause a bit of 'wind' and/or digestive discomfort in the early stages so best advice is to start slow with one tablespoon per day for a few days before increasing to two or three as your system becomes acclimatised.

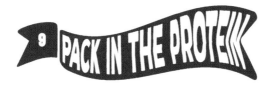

How much, how often and best sources are the 3 questions most debated currently when it comes to protein foods and protein-rich extras.

I continually encourage my readers and followers to sign up to my free newsletters and/or have a swatch at my blog and my Facebook page in order to keep up to date with diet news and when it comes to keeping up to date with the latest news on the protein front, this is important as the pendulum is swinging around like crazy. Some experts suggest that there is generally too much protein in our diets (particularly in Western diets), others fear that many of us are protein-deficient and then there are those that do little other than cause confusion by hitting us with the rather complex biochemical principles of how proteins work within the body and we are more often than not, none the wiser.

Here's the way I see it right now but as recommended, keep an eagle eye on my diet news as things may change and universal agreement may be a long way off! So for now, let's look at what we know where protein levels, cell strength and fat loss are concerned.

Protein is what holds us together and we need good levels on a daily basis to allow every single cell in our body and brain to repair and regenerate. Without it we suffer.

If we are largely sedentary most days, exercise doesn't play much of a role in our lives and we embark on a calorie-restricted diet we lose weight but way too often something like 20-30% of the weight lost is body weight rather than body fat and the loss of body weight means there is a strong chance we lose muscle. We may drop a dress/trouser size or two but we end up with skinny arms and legs and sagging skin and still have a fat belly which is likely not the look we are aiming for. We simply can't afford to lose lean muscle mass, we must concentrate on preserving or gaining it.

A POUND OF MUSCLE WEIGHS THE SAME AS A POUND OF FAT BUT MUSCLE TAKES UP A LOT LESS ROOM THAN FAT SO NOT ONLY DO WE LOOK LEANER AND FITTER BUT WE ALSO FEEL STRONGER, HAVE MORE ENERGY AND ARE A GREAT DEAL MORE LIKELY TO LOSE EXCESS BODY FAT FASTER.

Regular and relatively strenuous exercise alone is unlikely to result in desired fat loss, but combining a fitness-enhancing and muscle-building programme with a healthy and balanced diet is hard to argue against.

Recommendations regarding how much protein we should consume in a day dependent on how active we are and whose advice we choose to follow generally vary between 0.8g and 1.2g per kg of bodyweight but recent research suggests that if we exercise regularly and fairly strenuously (which is vital for heart, bone and immune health), these figures may be woefully short, particularly when endeavouring to lose excess body fat.

A number of studies indicate that a higher protein intake (between 1.5g and 2.2g per kg of bodyweight) coupled with a healthy weight loss diet and strenuous exercise 6 days per week results in both a greater increase in lean body mass and the loss of more fat than the same programmes providing less protein.

To work out your minimum and maximum daily protein intake, simply multiply your weight in kgs by 1.5 and 2.2 **but ensure that this is your healthy weight and not your current weight if you are carrying excess body fat.** This is very important!

A person currently weighing 65kg but whose lean and healthy weight should be 55kgs and is exercising regularly and strenuously would therefore require between 82g and 121g of protein per day and a person currently weighing 90kg but whose lean and healthy weight should be 75kg and is exercising regularly and strenuously would require between 112g and 165g of protein per day.

Your diet plan has been devised to provide around 100g of protein per day for three reasons. One, because there is substantial evidence that the health, energy-enhancing and protective benefits of increasing our intake beyond the recommended levels are persuasive, two, because higher levels of protein in every meal and snack spread over the day are associated with an increase in the release of the hormones which control hunger and cravings - big stumbling blocks for dieters - and three, because 100 is a nice easy number to work with!

Getting a bit more protein into your day is not just about eating more animal flesh and quaffing protein shakes! The list of foods that add protein to your day is hugely varied and many forget this. Here are the important ones - all of which are included in your diet plan:

red meats	quinoa and 'ancient grains'
poultry and game	nuts and seeds and their butters
fish and shellfish	beans, lentils and legumes
eggs	root vegetables
tofu	cruciferous vegetables
dairy and non-dairy milks	avocado and other fruits
yoghurts, cheeses and butter	

Should you add protein powders to up your intake? It kind of depends on your day and the size of your wallet! Like all supplements, they are supplementary to a good diet and should never be regarded as a replacement but having said that, there may be days when it's just not possible to factor in decent levels of protein so adding a 20g to 25g scoop of protein powder to a juice or smoothie has some merit but try not to make it a daily habit - real food is way more delicious and a great deal less pricey!

And… if you regularly go to the gym, are surrounded by 'protein shake devotees' and think you may be missing out, don't panic. Just make sure that your gym bag contains a protein-rich post workout snack and you will be wolfing down just as much, if not more protein than they have in their shakes and yours involves 'chewing' which encourages the early release of enzymes which promote improved digestion and increased satiety. A small pot of natural yoghurt or cottage cheese, a couple of oatcakes with almond butter and a crisp apple or a small tub of hummus, a bunch of vegetable sticks and a small pack of spiced nuts and seeds will do the trick!

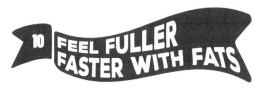

Fats in our diet are so important that they deserve a whole book but for now I am going to keep things simple and hope that by the end of just a couple of pages, you will be charging out to stock up!

Fats (both saturated and unsaturated) are vital to our health and as long as we steer well clear of the ones that have been chemically 'rearranged' or have been turned into fats that bear little or no resemblance to the natural plant and seed oils from whence they came through major 'processing' which makes them super-cheap to produce and gives them a shelf life that food producers love, they should play a important role in your diet and your life if you want to stay healthy, get slim and stay slim.

This is where I beg you to ignore the hundreds of pages on the internet from those who continue to advise that you 'limit your fats' and 'base your meals on fibre-rich starchy carbohydrates' - I have already covered the fat storing properties of starchy carbohydrates!

WHY ARE FATS SO IMPORTANT?

- They play a vital role in the health of our bones.
- They help us absorb fat-soluble nutrients found in various foods.
- They help to lower a substance in the blood that may increase our risk of heart disease.

- They help to protect us against harmful micro-organisms in the digestive tract.

- They help to improve our energy levels and lift our mood.

- They help to protect the liver from toxins.

- They help to boost our immune system.

- They play a vital role in the health of our brain, heart and nervous system.

- They help us reduce stored body fat by raising our metabolic rate.

- They help redress hormone imbalances.

- They have far-reaching anti-inflammatory benefits.

- They are rich in protective antioxidants.

- They help to protect us against mental decline.

- They have positive effects on fat burning and weight reduction.

- They are filling and taste great!

FATS INCLUDED IN YOUR DIET PLAN

fish and shellfish

olives and olive oil

avocados and avocado oil

coconut oil

nuts and seeds and their oils
and butters

sprouted beans and seeds

yoghurts, milks, cheese and butters

eggs

grass/pasture-fed animals and their products

poultry and game

beans, lentils and legumes

tofu, tempeh and other non-genetically-modified soy products

pumpkin and squash

dark green leafy vegetables

oats

6 Changes to Make Within 2 Weeks

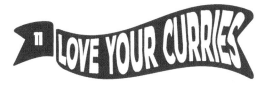

11 LOVE YOUR CURRIES

The notion that fat cells are simply a storage depot for body energy has now been irrefutably revised. Fat cells are actually very active and produce hormones that trigger metabolic processes in various different parts of the body. The hormones produced include oestradiol, a precursor which controls reproduction, leptin which controls appetite by binding to receptors in the brain, telling us when we are full and adiponectin which controls blood sugar levels by heightening the body's sensitivity to insulin, the hormone that ensures the sugars absorbed from our diet are ferried out of the bloodstream and put to work to assist in the generation of energy.

When we overeat, fat cells expand and if they are regularly over-stuffed (particularly those around the middle), inflammatory chemicals leap into action and interfere with the balance of the weight-controlling hormones. This can result is us becoming less sensitive to signals telling us we have had enough to eat so we eat more and our insulin response is dulled, creating increased episodes of hypoglycaemia (low blood sugar) which prompt us to reach for more food to counteract the tiredness, fuzzy brain, irritability and low mood that go with the territory.

Dieters often blame the desire to eat more on a lack of willpower and whilst desire plays a huge part in what, when and how much we eat, our biochemistry has a lot to answer for. The body will always do the very best it possibly can to ensure that homeostasis (balance) is maintained. Survival is its number one priority and no matter how often or seriously the balance is disrupted, it will continue to make adjustments to try to get things back on track.

Ballooning fat cells caused by overeating are not the only reason the inflammatory chemicals are stimulated - another major cause is what we actually eat. The altered fats found in deep-fried, fast, processed and junk foods and foods with crazy levels of added sugars which invade many diets are the chief culprits here.

But let's focus on the foods that minimise the likelihood of inflammation and enable the weight-controlling hormones to do what they do best; control our appetite and encourage efficient blood sugar management. These include vegetables, fruits, oily fish, nuts and seeds and their oils, whole grains and herbs and spices.

Herbs and spices are particularly important because they are very rich in antioxidants, substances that protect body cells from the damage created when the inflammatory process is in full swing.

The antioxidant-rich, anti-inflammatory properties of herbs and spices encourage fat burning whilst reducing fat storage.

They also add flavour to food which results in reduced salt consumption - too much salt prompts fluid retention, another fat loss adversary.

But, what about the perceived metabolism-boosting attributes of herbs and spices when it comes to turning up body heat and increasing the pace at which we burn calories and lose weight? There is strong evidence that a diet which regularly includes hot spices and pungent herbs provides us with a neat little advantage on the fat burning front so if you 'like it hot', go for it!

Here are the front-running, fat busting and health-protective herbs and spices (a great many of which are included in your diet plan).

chillies	cardamom	mustard
cinnamon	cloves	sage
black pepper	cumin	oregano
cayenne/ground chilli	ginger	turmeric
	marjoram	thyme

A FEW WORDS OF ADVICE HOWEVER...

Steer clear of curries and highly spiced or herbed dishes that are overly-creamy or buttery.

Create your own dishes wherever possible, use the freshest herbs and spices you can find and buy them as you need them rather than 'stocking up' and letting them sit on a shelf or in a drawer for months on end where they will lose a deal of their intensity and thermogenic powers.

Whilst following the 2 week diet plan, stick with my herby and spicy meal and snack recipes and recommendations.

Make rice and noodles an occasional and small addition to your meals and forget naans, chapatis and parathas.

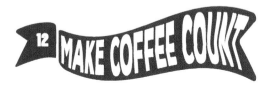

Continuing on the subject of boosting metabolism in a bid to lose weight faster, here's the latest news on coffee. There is evidence that it may be a valued helper.

Bodybuilders and athletes have been using caffeine to reduce body fat for over 20 years but it is only recently that its fat-burning properties have been further investigated. It's all about the what, the when and the how but it seems that deprivation of our morning cuppa doesn't have to be on the cards!

Properly used, caffeine stimulates the central nervous system, increases the use of body fat as fuel and preserves glycogen levels (the glucose stored in the liver and muscles). It is also a diuretic so it promotes the loss of water from our body cells and raises body temperature, so we overheat and our metabolic rate increases.

Studies focused on professional athletes reveal that caffeine taken up to 3 hours prior to training allow them to perform both longer and harder before exhaustion and increase the use of fat for fuel, thereby sparing the glycogen stored in their muscles which, when depleted causes what is commonly known as *hitting the wall* where energy levels take a major dive and more glucose-rich foods and drinks have to be consumed to enable them to continue.

But, few of us are professional athletes so can caffeine play a role in fat burning for us amateurs? Yes. Caffeine increases the number of calories the body burns at rest. A single 100mg dose of caffeine may increase our metabolic rate by 3-4% for at least an hour and a half afterwards. 100mg consumed every two hours for 12 hours has also been shown to increase our daily metabolic rate by 8-11% (one cup of reasonably strong coffee contains anywhere between 65mg and 115mg of caffeine). However, it doesn't have the same effect in everyone.

One study compared the effects of caffeine in 10 lean and 10 obese women. The rise in metabolic rate following the consumption of caffeine was just under 5% in the obese women and just over 7% in the lean women and although the effects of the caffeine on the metabolic rate could no longer be seen the following day, both groups were still burning between 10% and 30% more fat at rest than before the caffeine trial.

I am not, however encouraging a cup of coffee every 2 hours over a 12 hour period! Coffee has rather many downsides:

- Many of the chemicals in coffee irritate the stomach lining causing an increase of stomach acid leading to digestive disorders.

- It may raise blood pressure.

- It may interfere with our sleep quality.

- It may cause problems with blood sugar control.

- It excites more rapid peristaltic movements of the intestines resulting in shortened transit times and less absorption of nutrients.

- It stimulates more frequent urination and subsequent loss of various vitamins and minerals.

- It may leach calcium from the bones increasing the risk of osteoporosis.

However, caffeine does have a role to play in fat loss. When used in conjunction with a healthy diet and lifestyle it can make losing fat a little faster and a little easier, particularly when consumed before exercise.

So if you want to give it a go, here's the plan: Have a double espresso or a small cup of strong filtered coffee first thing in the morning (no milk or sugar), exercise for 30-45 minutes and have a large glass of water when you get back to base. If you are unable to exercise until later in the day, do the same but as many find caffeine can disrupt their sleep pattern when consumed in the 4 to 6 hours before bed, best advice is to follow this recommendation only on days when you are able to exercise earlier in the day.

If you don't like coffee, you may wish to experiment with caffeine tablets (1 x 100mg before exercise) or have a small, strong cup of green tea which has a similar but less powerful effect as it contains only around a third of the caffeine of a cup of strong coffee.

IMPORTANT!

Whatever you do, please don't resort to caffeinated fizzy drinks like *Coca Cola* or *Red Bull* in a bid to boost your caffeine levels and increase fat burning. As mentioned previously, the full sugar versions are groaning with added sugars and the diet versions are groaning with health-disrupting artificial sweeteners and chemicals and have no place in the fat loss game.

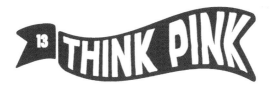

The pigment responsible for giving salmon, shrimps, prawns, langoustine, crabs and lobster their pink colour when cooked is a plant chemical called astaxanthin which is synthesised as a direct result of the microalgae they feed on. Research suggests that this naturally-occurring plant chemical may be the most powerful antioxidant to go under the microscope thus far and has been shown to provide the body with an internal sunscreen, protecting us from the damaging effects of UV rays from the sun. Small amounts of UV light are beneficial as it enables the body to make Vitamin D which aids in the absorption of calcium, helping to form and maintain strong bones but few are unaware that over-exposure contributes to prematurely ageing skin and in some cases skin cancer. This exciting discovery has already led to astaxanthin being included in anti-ageing skin care products and sunscreens.

Furthermore, because astaxanthin has been proven to efficiently cross the blood-brain barrier, it offers protection to the brain, the central nervous system and the eyes.

It has also been shown to increase the usage of fat as an energy source and accelerate fat burning during exercise.

A group of Japanese researchers recently demonstrated that mice given astaxanthin along with a relatively high fat diet had significantly lower body weight and body fat levels compared to mice fed on a similar diet of a similar calorie count without the addition of astaxanthin. In another study, mice were given astaxanthin along with a daily exercise routine. After four weeks the animals were placed on a treadmill to test a range of physical parameters and fat usage during exercise was increased. At present, no human studies have been concluded but researchers are confident that this powerful substance may play an important role in the fight against our globally-increasing waistlines.

There is another reason why astaxanthin is a valuable addition to a diet focused on fat loss; its anti-inflammatory properties. As discussed previously, inflammation is no friend where fat loss is the goal and it is astaxanthin's role in good gastric health that is important here. Inflammation in the 21st century gut is on the increase and a condition known as *leaky gut syndrome* is largely to blame.

The digestive tract consists of a long tube, which connects the mouth to the anus. After food is swallowed it passes through the oesophagus to the stomach, where it is churned up with acid and broken down into tiny particles by stomach enzymes. These then pass into the small intestine which is around 20 feet long and its major function is to digest and absorb the valuable nutrients from the food particles that arrive from the stomach before releasing them into the bloodstream. Then it's off to the liver for further processing to produce the essentials which are quickly delivered to body cells to generate the energy to make new cells, repair cells that are worn out and generally keep us in good health.

The inner lining of the small intestine can however, become inflamed due to infection, because of toxic substances within foods or as a result of the over-consumption of processed fats, sugars and food additives which over time weaken its permeability. When the gut becomes *leaky*, overly-large and damaging food molecules enter the bloodstream causing an immediate response by the immune system which recognises these invaders as a threat to health. As they pass through the liver they have to be detoxified to limit the potential damage but this places an enormous burden on the liver, stressing its detoxification capabilities and resulting in these substances being only partially processed and/or allowed to build up. In a bid to restore its health and efficiency and prevent these partially-processed toxins from being released back into the bloodstream, the liver is forced to pack them up and send them off for safe storage and our fat cells are only too willing to accommodate!

Frustratingly, it is hard enough to encourage fat cells to release their energy and shrink because they are programmed to store fat for survival but it is even harder when they are storing toxins which when released into the bloodstream are likely to create havoc and compromise our health. This is damage limitation at its best but can be a major stumbling block when we want to shift fat.

Fat loss becomes a whole lot easier, quicker and more maintainable in the long term when the cells that line the small intestine are healthy and strong.

Astaxanthin has not only shown itself to be protective of the outer membranes of these cells, reducing the chance of toxic substances compromising their permeability but also has the ability to mount an impressive anti-inflammatory effect should toxic substances sneak through into the bloodstream. **This is clearly a substance that is earning its stripes as a fat loss warrior.**

I am well-aware that this tip that will have varied appeal. Some of you don't like or don't eat seafood, some have allergies to certain or all shellfish but if you are a fan, I urge you to factor a 'portion of pink' into your day as often as possible - it is remarkably easy and because these 'swimmers' are a rich source of protein and fats, you don't need much to stem your hunger. And along the way you are getting a good dose of health-enhancing Omega fats and health-protective astaxanthin! Alternatively, you may wish to consider supplementing (see recommended products).

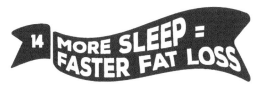

A number of studies have found that those who get less than 6 hours of sleep per night tend to gain more weight over time than people who get 7 to 8 hours or more.

The production of two hormones, leptin and ghrelin which control hunger and fullness are influenced by how much or how little sleep we get. Leptin controls appetite, is produced by the fat cells and tells the brain when energy stores are replenished and we have had enough to eat. Ghrelin controls hunger, is produced in the stomach and tells the brain when we are hungry and need nourishment. When these hormones are working optimally we are better able to control when we eat and how much we eat but unfortunately they are easily disrupted. If the signals to the brain are scrambled it is all too easy to just go along with our desires resulting in us gorging rather than grazing and likely weight gain.

Leptin levels peak when we are asleep so if we don't get enough sleep, levels drop and if we are regularly deprived, they stay depressed and the brain interprets this as a reduction in energy stores prompting us to eat more in an effort to get the balance back. Continued lack of sleep also causes ghrelin levels to rise, which means our appetite is regularly stimulated and we want more food. The two combined set the stage for overeating so clearly, getting our eight hours a night is critical.

But, what if you are one of the millions for whom a good night's sleep is the goal but rarely a reality? You either can't get to sleep and toss and turn for hours or you wake in the middle of the night and can't get back to sleep; your leptin and ghrelin levels are likely all over the place and fat loss isn't going to be easy, so what can you do?

Have a bedtime snack that includes foods that encourage the production of the happy and relaxed neurotransmitter, serotonin which in turn, promotes the release of the sleep-inducing hormone, melatonin. When you are trying to shift fat, the suggestion that you should eat before you go to bed sits uncomfortably with many but when you understand that sleep deprivation promotes weight gain and balanced blood sugar levels and a good night's sleep aid weight loss you may wish to reconsider.

Serotonin levels are to a degree, linked to the amount of tryptophan (an essential amino acid found in protein foods) in the blood and as blood and brain levels of tryptophan rise and fall, so do levels of serotonin. Tryptophan can be the runt of the litter when it comes to competing with the other amino acids to get from the bloodstream into the brain, but a little starch added to a protein-rich snack creates a diversion allowing tryptophan to take the stage.

SO HERE'S THE PLAN...

For at least a couple of nights before you embark on your diet plan and for as many nights as you possibly can manage during the first two weeks, go to bed 60 to 90 minutes earlier than usual, make the room as dark as possible (wear an eye mask if necessary), ensure you are neither too hot nor too cold, don't watch TV in bed or read or text or email or check your Facebook page, settle down to go to sleep and if your brain refuses to stop buzzing, listen to some calming music or one of the many sleep-inducing apps available for download.

Set your alarm for exactly the time you need to get up and when it goes off, get up immediately and open the curtains/blinds - do not press the snooze button!

Should you find during the first few days that even when employing all of the above strategies, you still can't get to sleep, have a **bedtime snack** 20 minutes before you get ready for bed and/or if you wake in the middle of the night and struggle to get back to sleep, keep one of the suggested **bedside snacks** within reach and hoover it down before settling back down. **You will find all the bedtime and bedside snack recommendations in your diet plan/recipes.**

Why total darkness for sleep and bright daylight first thing in the morning? To optimally-manage your melatonin levels. These rise during the hours of darkness so the possibility of restful sleep is increased and fall in bright light so you start the day full of energy rather than feeling sluggish.

Of course, it is all a great deal simpler in theory than it ever is in practice, particularly for those of you who are habitual night birds but as a good night's sleep on a regular basis is so very important not only to the avoidance of debilitating health conditions but also to successful fat loss, I urge you to treat this tip as a priority and do everything you can to get a good sleep habit going.

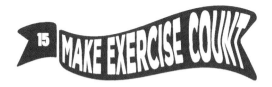

Many adopt the 'zero to hero' approach when they decide the time has come to lose weight and get fitter and from a standing start of doing little or no exercise on a weekly basis are suddenly donning the running shoes or gym kit and throwing themselves into an intensive programme on a daily basis. And there's nothing wrong with that... except for a couple of things. Firstly, it's not in the least bit uncommon for injury to strike when you dive in a little too enthusiastically as body tissues may not be 'ready' or capable of absorbing the new 'forces' and injury can seriously hamper your efforts. Secondly, if you want to see faster fitness results alongside faster fat loss, the type of programme you adopt is important - some work better than others.

I am not an expert in the fitness department, although I do have a qualification in Sports Nutrition but I try to keep right up to date with the latest recommendations of 'those in the know', follow their advice as far as my own personal fitness is concerned and because I have limited time in which to fit exercise into my day, am more than happy to pass on their words of wisdom to my readers, many of whom may also struggle time-wise.

Here's what *Ben Camara*, owner of No1 Fitness **no1fitness.co.uk** whose knowledge, passion and expertise have helped countless clients, including many celebrities, recommends...

RESISTANCE TRAINING

To emphasise muscle definition and reduce body fat in the most time-efficient way, quality over quantity is the key. You train hard but for a shorter time and fat burning is accelerated because there is an increased secretion of both growth hormone and noradrenalin, two hormones that help to mobilise fat stores and use fat for fuel. More calories are expended both during the intense workout and because your BMR (basal metabolic rate) is increased for many hours after you have finished training - that's when the fat burning kicks in.

By using dumbbells, exercise machines, your own body weight, bottles of water, elastic tubing, ankle and wrist weights or exercise bricks, muscles are strengthened by pitting each group against a force (resistance). To develop a muscle you must work all the fibres within it which means pushing them to their limit for short periods of time, resting them briefly then repeating the process. You work with a weight that is heavy enough so that the last few repetitions become difficult to perform (this is not the kind of exercise where you chat to a friend while you work out - it requires concentration and determination). When a muscle is overloaded, lactic acid is produced causing the 'burn' in the muscle that ultimately leads to muscular fatigue - you have to push past that sensation and ensure your mind doesn't give up before your body. The rest between repetitions enables the lactic acid to be flushed from the bloodstream, allowing the muscles to be refreshed before working them again.

Recommendations vary but generally 45 to 55 minutes, 3 to 4 times a week is a good goal. To allow the muscles to repair and regenerate 48 hours should be allowed between sessions. This enables protein synthesis to take place (the process by which the body repairs muscle tissue) preventing injury. However, if you adopt a programme where you work different muscle areas on different days, a shorter rest period is quite acceptable.

AND IT'S NEVER TOO LATE TO START.

In one study of elderly men and women (average age 87) who lifted weights three times a week for ten weeks, base muscle strength increased by a staggering 113% on average. This improvement enabled them to walk 12% faster than before, climb 28% more stairs and in a notable number of cases, lose excess body fat.

INTERVAL TRAINING

Whilst resistance training is the most effective for fat burning for many hours after a workout, it should be coupled with aerobic exercise for a number of reasons.

The cardiovascular system becomes more efficient at delivering oxygen to working muscle, delaying the lactic acid build-up which allows you to train at a higher level of intensity. Aerobic exercise also expands the network of blood vessels that allow nutrients to be absorbed into body tissues and the more capillaries we have the better the body becomes at utilising the nutrients for muscular repair. This expanded network of blood vessels also helps to clear waste products, particularly carbon dioxide from the food burning process. Efficient exchange of oxygen and nutrients in and carbon dioxide and waste out is paramount for fit and healthy body tissue.

In addition, the mitochondria (the energy factories) expand in size and number and require more energy. Once they have used up the glycogen (the stored glucose within the muscle cells and the liver), they call on the fat cells to release energy. Interval training provides significant benefits over steady state exercise and is more effective at 'burning' fat because as with resistance training, the fat burning is prolonged after activity. This type of training involves intense effort for one minute followed by less intense effort for between one and four minutes. During the intense phase the lactic acid builds up quickly and during the less intense phase it is cleared from the blood and oxygen stores are replenished. This is repeated multiple times.

HERE'S AN EXAMPLE

If you are a jogger, run as fast and as hard as you can for one minute then reduce your speed to a steady jog for between one and four minutes. Keep repeating until your 30 minutes is up. The same applies to rowing, cycling, swimming, skipping, using a mini trampoline or whatever gets your heart pumping. If you are on the treadmill in the gym, turn the knob to as fast as you can cope with for one minute then turn the speed down to a manageable jog for four minutes. A mere five repetitions and your 30 minutes of cardio are done! As you get fitter you can reduce the number of minutes between the intense phases to two minutes or even one minute during the middle section of your workout.

Resistance training for 45 to 55 minutes on Monday, Wednesday and Friday (or Tuesday, Thursday and Saturday) and Interval Training for 30 minutes on the other three days with one day of rest suits many peoples' timetables, but you may prefer to do both in a longer workout three times a week with one rest day between each.

WHICH SHOULD YOU DO FIRST?

Resistance followed by Interval appears to have the edge. Since the body's preferred energy source is glucose that's what we should target first. Resistance Training does that. The body uses the glucose from recently consumed carbohydrates in the bloodstream followed by the stored glucose in the muscles and liver when we perform any type of anaerobic exercise. Resistance Training is anaerobic - it uses minimal oxygen and as fat can only be burned in the presence of oxygen the fat cells won't be mobilised into releasing their energy stores until after we stop. By the time we embark on the Interval Training, glycogen stores are pretty well used up and because Interval Training is aerobic (uses lots of oxygen) the body will have to call on the fat stores for energy. And, because of the intensity of both sessions the body will continue to burn calories for hours afterwards, requiring fat stores to continue providing some or much of that energy.

UNFIT OR UNUSED TO EXERCISE?

Don't worry, the principles of Resistance Training and Interval Training apply no matter where you start. Resistance Training is all about introducing some weights into your life and if you want to start with a couple of cans of baked beans you will still be creating 'the force' and within a couple of weeks you can raise your game and seek out the litre bottles of water. From there it's all uphill. Similarly, Interval Training is all about moving as fast as you can manage for one minute followed by one to four minutes of slowing the pace. Walking is a great way to start - brisk for one minute, less intense for one to four minutes. As you get fitter, your body will become acclimatised and you can push the intensity.

NB: If you want to see great and long-lasting results from the above well-researched exercise combination to find the fit, lean and toned body you know is lurking somewhere under those excess pounds of flesh, you may wish to delve more deeply into the science. If so, read some of the many studies available, buy a book that covers this type of programme in detail or enlist the services of a personal trainer who practices these principles.

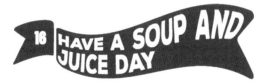
16 HAVE A SOUP AND JUICE DAY

This is a tip/change that may **not** suit everyone but I am determined to include it!

What I am suggesting is that once or twice a week both during your 2 week diet plan and thereafter on a regular basis, you give your digestion a bit of *time out* and hike the fat burning up a little by concentrating on nourishing soups, juices and smoothies and factoring in a **14 hour 'no eating' window**.

Let me be crystal clear here. It is **not** a purely liquid day and it is **not** simply another way of encouraging you to jump on the currently-popular intermittent fasting bandwagon. The soups and juices I recommend are gutsy and often require a spoon or fork and the 14 hour 'no eating' window simply means you have your last meal of the day a little earlier than you do normally, skip breakfast and have your first soup, juice or smoothie of the day around mid morning.

The reason I include this tip is because many who are overweight and decide to embark on a fat loss plan already suffer from poor or inefficient digestion and this can hamper your efforts. Whether it be bloating, wind, heartburn, IBS or simply general tiredness, the digestive system has a lot to answer for when it is not working at its best so giving it an easy day every now and then can sharpen things up nicely.

The goal is to ensure that the soups, juices and smoothies are tasty and filling and provide a wealth of nutrients so you still have the energy to get through your day, but involve no gut irritation and the **14 hour no food window** allows the gut to rest, calm things down and repair. And a rather pleasing side-effect is that your Soup and Juice Day presents your liver (one of the hardest-working organs in the body) with an opportunity to crack on with processing and eliminating the toxic waste that may have built up over time and enable it to spend a little more time on fat-burning!

If you decide to follow this suggestion, you will find all the details of how to plan ahead for a Soup and Juice Day in your diet plan.

IMPORTANT!

I recommend three Soup and Juice Days during the 2 weeks with three days between each where you follow the diet plan but should you decide to do a few Soup and Juice Days in a row, you need not worry about becoming under-nourished. My advice however, is to only embark on this route if your timetable is not too frantic as you may feel a bit below par, headachy, cold etc as your liver and digestive system get to grips with the change in pace over a few days. Don't be tempted to do any longer than a few days at a time - you will quickly become bored and diet variety is paramount for successful fat loss both in the short term and in the long term!

THE SECRET TO A SUCCESSFUL SOUP AND JUICE DAY IS TO PLAN AHEAD!

4 Changes to Make as you Move Forward

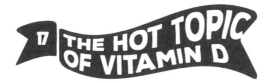

THE HOT TOPIC OF VITAMIN D

Not another epidemic to get our heads around? I hear you ask. I'm afraid so! Vitamin D deficiency has now reached epidemic levels with recent estimates indicating that more than 50% of the global population is at risk. A high prevalence of vitamin D deficiency has been found across all age groups in all populations studied and even those who are otherwise healthy are not immune.

So where did it go so horribly wrong? Well, it's not really news, it's just that more money is being spent on research and the findings are not too sunny. Vitamin D is produced by our skin when we are in strong sunlight and studies of traditional people living in East Africa give us a few clues as to what was probably 'normal' when we first appeared on the planet. These people all have dark skin which gives them built-in sun protection, spend most of the day outdoors but seek shade whenever possible. Their skin and sun habits are similar to our ancestors who lived in the same environment but as we moved north to colder climates we weren't exposed to the same levels of strong sunlight, our skin became paler and vitamin D levels dropped. However, for centuries we still spent a great deal of time working outdoors and even in many of the most northern parts of the globe we ate a lot of fish, the richest food source of vitamin D.

But as industrialisation flourished and technology developed, the pale amongst us increasingly worked indoors and after a long working day spent what few hours were left of the day settling in front of a warming fire and sadly fish didn't feature as often in our diets. And then came sunscreens. Skin cancer was on the rise and governments and health experts ensured that we all became critically aware of the dangers of unprotected sun exposure. Valid advice but like so many health scares - over-asserted. In a matter of only a few years we were suddenly lathering tub-loads of factor 20, 30 or 50 on our pale skins and making our *little darlings* wear garish and highly-protective clothing on the beach whilst their southern counterparts were running around with little or no clothes on. Cynical perhaps but true!

A number of studies indicate that muslim women who wear burka have amongst the highest levels of deficiency even when vitamin D-rich foods are included in their diet. And interestingly, a huge percentage of the research into vitamin D deficiency has been undertaken in Scandinavian countries where hours of sunlight from November to March are woefully short and most of these countries promote regular consumption of vitamin D-enriched milk in an effort to make up for the shortfall.

Vitamin D is actually a hormone rather than a vitamin and understanding this is important. Hormones are produced naturally within the body, vitamins must be obtained through our diet. The body can make most of the vitamin D it needs as long as we get sunshine into our lives - the action of sunlight on our skin produces a substance which is converted by the liver to yet another substance then further converted in the kidneys to the active and usable form of vitamin D. Daily consumption of D-rich foods or D-fortified foods increase levels. However the above statistics indicate that this is not happening and the health risks associated with D-deficiency are wide ranging; brittle bones, muscle weakness, mental decline, high blood pressure, auto-immune conditions, cancers... the list is growing.

SO WHAT ABOUT VITAMIN D AND FAT LOSS?

Vitamin D deficiency has been shown to disrupt the delicate balance of insulin production by the pancreas and increase the possibility of insulin resistance which over time leads not only to weight gain but also an increased risk of type 2 diabetes. Research indicates that women who are D-deficient carry between 40% and 80% more abdominal fat than their D-rich counterparts and this is largely because fat cells are not just storage depots; **they are metabolically active and vitamin D, which is stored in fat cells has an important role to play in regulating how much fat we store and how much we burn.** Leptin, the hormone that controls appetite is produced by the fat cells and tells the brain when energy stores are replenished and we have had enough to eat but it appears that vitamin D deficiency can interfere with this appetite-suppressing hormone causing us to eat more.

Because vitamin D is stored in fat cells, one would imagine that the bigger our fat cells, the more vitamin D we are able to store, allowing its release into the bloodstream for bone building and cellular health but quite the opposite has been noted. The fatter we are, the higher our risk of deficiency because vitamin D gets locked inside fat cells and unavailable for use. In one study, a group of obese adults (BMI above 30) and a group of lean adults (BMI of 19-24) were exposed to the same amount of UVA/UVB rays and blood levels of vitamin D in the lean adults rose by almost double those in their obese counterparts indicating that when we are overweight we need a lot more.

SO WHAT CAN YOU DO?

We know that vitamin D is primarily synthesised in the skin after exposure to sunshine and it was previously thought that as little as 5-10 minutes of sun exposure on arms, legs and face three times a week without sunscreen between 11am and 2pm during the spring, summer, and autumn should provide a light-skinned individual with adequate vitamin D and allow for some storage of any excess for use during the colder, darker months with minimal risk of skin damage - those with dark skin may require twice or three times the exposure. However, a recent study was set up to assess how much vitamin D is needed to ensure optimal rather than just adequate levels in the average person and found that a minimum of 4,000IU of vitamin D is required daily to maintain optimal blood levels. 3,500 men and women had their vitamin D levels measured and completed online surveys to monitor vitamin D status and health outcomes over five years. The researchers found that daily intakes of between 4000IU and 8000IU are needed to maintain blood levels of vitamin D needed to effectively reduce the risk of disease and importantly they also found that this dose was very safe.

So, from a health and fat loss point of view, daily exposure of your skin to sunlight and a diet packed with foods rich in vitamin D (oily fish - particularly salmon, eggs, mushrooms, butter and milk products) are crucial. You may also wish to have your D levels checked. A simple blood test available at your doctor's surgery measures the level of 25 hydroxy-vitamin D, the chemical formed in the liver during the process that converts sunlight into vitamin D and if the sunshine and the D-rich foods don't see you reaching the mark, supplementation may be required.

IF SUPPLEMENTING, ALWAYS OPT FOR VITAMIN D3 CHOLECALCIFEROL

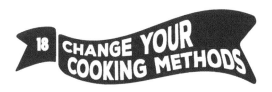

18 CHANGE YOUR COOKING METHODS

A healthy, fat loss diet plan should always include a variety of foods. Foods that offer exceptional properties, foods that offer and retain vitamins, minerals and plant chemicals that are going to prompt improved energy levels, a stronger immune system, a healthier body, a sharper brain plus weight loss and weight maintenance... but how you prepare and cook them is as important as the foods involved.

Wherever possible, buy the freshest foods in as natural a state as possible.

TOP TIP: keep an eye on the discounted shelves which offer foods that are perilously close to their 'sell by' date. The freshest foods have the shortest shelf life simply because they are largely devoid of preservatives so grab them and reap the benefits!

Going raw and lightly steaming your food are the very best ways to retain freshness and maximise on all-round nourishment. Roasting, baking and microwaving are also good cooking methods. Even barbecuing can be 'healthy' as long as you do it right (ie: don't have the 'fire' raging hot and cremate the food!)

So what about sautéing and shallow frying? It's all about using the right oils and butters. As discussed in **Feel Fuller Faster with Fats**, naturally-occurring fats are vital to good health and successful fat loss, cheap, 'fake' and overly-processed fats make us sick and fat.

And when it comes to using fats and oils in our cooking, there are a few very important things to remember:

• *The 'vegetable oils' that line the supermarket shelves, sit there for weeks on end, come in clear plastic bottles (and are therefore subject to oxidation) and are marketed as being 'healthy' are not. In addition to having already been through a great deal of processing which leaves them feebly-short of health-enhancing properties, when heated and used in cooking, they release toxic chemicals known as aldehydes which have been linked to cancers, heart disease and dementia.*

- *All liquid fats are very easily damaged, turning them quickly from being health-promoting to potentially health-damaging so even the very best, cold-pressed and minimally-processed must be treated with great care and not allowed to overheat or 'smoke'.*

- *Unrefined hard (solid at room temperature) fats like butter, ghee, lard, tallow and coconut oil are less easily damaged by heat because of their molecular structure.*

- *Some oils should never be exposed to heat but rather drizzled over cooked foods and dishes before being served.*

The selection of oils now available is bewildering to say the least and it can be very tempting to keep an impressive collection in stock. However, they have short lives. The best, which should always be in dark glass bottles and kept in a cool, dark place or in the fridge won't retain their goodness for much longer than a month or so.

BEST OILS AND BUTTERS FOR COOKING

Avocado Oil - unrefined, cold-pressed and where possible, organic

Coconut Oil - unrefined, 'virgin', cold-pressed and where possible, organic

Olive Oil - unrefined, cold-pressed and 'light' rather than 'extra virgin'

Grapeseed Oil - unrefined, cold-pressed and where possible, organic

Butter, Ghee, Lard and Tallow - from grass/pasture-fed animals

All the above don't become damaged when heated but should not be allowed to 'smoke'. They are also rich in important monounsaturated fats and offer good levels of vital nutrients.

BEST OILS AND BUTTERS FOR ADDING TO RAW AND LIGHTLY-COOKED FOODS

Avocado Oil - unrefined, cold-pressed and where possible, organic

Extra Virgin Olive Oil - cold-pressed and where possible, organic

Nut and Seed Oils - unrefined, cold-pressed and where possible, organic

Butter - from grass/pasture-fed animals

Nut and Seed Butters - sugar-free and where possible, organic

WHICH OILS AND BUTTERS ARE IN MY FRIDGE?

Being crucially-aware of the short life of all oils and butters, I tend to stock only a few (and occasionally add a few others dependent on what I am planning to cook). Here are my 'regulars':

Avocado Oil - for sautéing, light frying and stir frying, for roasting, for drizzling over steamed vegetables, soups, curries, casseroles and one-pot dishes after cooking, for adding to juices and smoothies and for use in dips

Light Olive Oil - for sautéing, light frying, stir frying and roasting

Extra Virgin Olive Oil - for drizzling over steamed vegetables, soups, curries, casseroles and one-pot dishes after cooking and for use in dips, dressings and minimally-cooked sauces

Coconut Oil - for sautéing, light frying, stir frying and roasting (and for my skin, hair and nails!)

Really Good Butter from Grass/Pasture-Fed Animals - for sautéing and light frying (always with the addition of a splash of avocado or light olive oil), for melting over lightly-cooked vegetables and for spreading

Flaxseed Oil - for drizzling over steamed vegetables, soups, curries, casseroles and one-pot dishes after cooking and for use in juices, smoothies, dips, dressings and minimally-cooked sauces. I am also rather partial to walnut oil, macadamia nut oil and the 'liquid gold', sympathetically-grown, harvested and lightly cold-pressed rapeseed oil from the McKenzie family farm in beautiful Perthshire in Scotland **www.cullisse.com**

Sugar-Free, Organic Almond Butter - for adding to curries and casseroles just before the end of cooking, for spreading on toast or crisp breads, for adding a bit more protein to a smoothie or simply to be eaten by the spoonful! I love and use all kinds of nut and seed butters but almond has to be my number one!

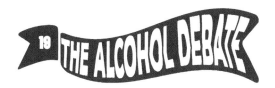

THE ALCOHOL DEBATE

There is some evidence that consumption of two to four glasses of red wine a day reduces the risk of a heart attack by up to an astonishing 32% due to the protective combination of the alcohol and resveratrol (and a few other plant chemicals therein). Music to the ears of all who are partial to the occasional glass or two! So can the odd tipple feature in a fat loss diet? In some cases, yes. It has a lot to do with what we drink, when we drink, how much we drink and what we eat before, during and after a glass of our favourite tipple!

There are two very important points to stress here. One is that if you don't currently drink alcohol, don't for heavens' sake take it up in a bid to cut your risk of heart disease - a healthy diet and lifestyle will take care of that (same applies to infrequent drinkers). Secondly, if you are a heavy drinker or alcohol plays a major part in your life, you are at risk of potentially serious health problems so you should make every effort to get consumption under control.

However, people who drink moderately (max 2 units per day for men, 1 unit for women) and are able to control their consumption (spread over the week as opposed to bingeing at the weekend) and don't have any of the absolute reasons why they shouldn't be drinking alcohol (pregnancy, breastfeeding, on medication, operating heavy machinery, poor health history, under age etc) can take comfort in the fact that while they are enjoying some down-time with glass in hand, there may be a few benefits!

Its heart-friendly properties are not the only benefit. A number of studies have found that adults with moderate alcohol intakes are at a lower risk of developing type 2 diabetes than adults who don't partake and analysis of some 15 studies concluded that moderate consumption may reduce the risk by around 30%. It has been suggested that this may be associated with improved insulin sensitivity.

So, how can you reap a few health benefits and enjoy the odd glass whilst following a fat loss program?

Best advice is to have an occasional glass of good red wine with your evening meal (Cabernet Sauvignon, Pinot Noir and Merlot are richest in protective plant chemicals). If your social life involves dining out, meeting friends/colleagues for a drink or entertaining at home, here are a few tips that can minimise the addition of calories without meaning you have to say "no" to invitations:

- Alcohol raises blood sugar very quickly, so always have a protein-rich snack before or with a drink (a couple of oatcakes with nut butter, a small pot of live natural yoghurt with fresh fruit, a chicken leg, a cold boiled egg, some crunchy baby vegetables with a small pot of hummus, a handful of almonds) to moderate the sugar spike.

- Alcohol dehydrates, so for every drink you have, have two large glasses of water; you will have to go to the ladies/mens room more often but you will seriously cut down on the amount of alcohol you consume. And, have a few glasses of water before bed (and keep another one by the bed) to help re-hydrate and ensure you feel fresh the next morning.

- Alcohol increases your appetite, lessens your resolve and removes inhibitions (!!!) so always make sure you have a friend/ partner around to keep you on track.

- Avoid fizzy mixers at all costs - they are full of sugar and the diet alternatives are no better, they just increase your desire for more sugar and consequently more alcohol.

- Avoid all lite beers, alcopops and ready-mixed spirit-based cocktails - sugar, sugar and yet more sugar!

- Aim for good quality wine, spirits on the rocks or with natural unsweetened fruit juice.

- Cocktails can be dangerous and are often high in sugar, but if you stick to Breezes, Martinis, Sours, Manhattans, Screwdrivers, Punches and Pimms (no sugar added, just the sweetness from the fruit), you shouldn't get into too much trouble. And, don't forget the nutritious, satisfying and delicious Bloody Mary or Bloody Caesar!

- Mix white wine with soda water to make it last twice as long and half the calories. If you can't bear to dilute it, opt for dry whites as these contain fewer calories than sweeter wines.

- Follow in the footsteps of celebrities and enjoy a glass of bubbly if funds allow. In general you drink less as it's served in smaller glasses and the bubbles fill you up.

- Most measures of spirits poured at home are larger than those served in bars and pubs with the result that your drink will probably contain twice as many calories. If you're going to do a lot of entertaining at home, it's worth investing in a spirits measure. Also, always pour spirits into the glass before adding ice or mixers, so you can actually see just how much alcohol is involved.

- Steer clear of beer, lager and cider as they're loaded with calories. And the higher the alcohol content, the more calories they contain. For example, a pint of standard beer contains around 160 calories, whereas a bottle of strong lager can contain more like 200 calories.

- Beware of trendy wine bars. Many serve spirits in double measures as the standard with the result that you get double the calories. Some pubs also serve 35ml measures of spirits rather than 25ml measures and so also contain more calories. Finally, watch out for huge wine glasses - some are so large that a glass of wine may actually be close to quarter of a bottle.

- Avoid creamy liqueurs after dinner and instead have a single shot of brandy if you really fancy ending your meal in style. Most cream-based liqueurs contain around 80-100 calories per 25ml measure compared with 50 calories in a single brandy.

- Remember that happy hours are designed to get you to drink more and keep you in the same place all night. Unfortunately, this means while the bar gains pounds, so do you as you indulge in far more drinks than you normally would.

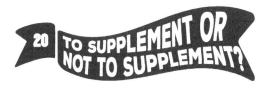

20 TO SUPPLEMENT OR NOT TO SUPPLEMENT?

Once broken down into their component parts, it is the carbohydrates, proteins and fats that we consume through our diet that not only help to generate the energy each and every body and brain cell requires to keep them 'alive and kicking' but also to provide the building blocks for their ongoing repair and regeneration.

This involves trillions of inordinately complex biochemical reactions which take place around the clock, every day of our lives and in the majority of cases, these reactions require certain vitamins and minerals to keep the big wheel turning.

SOME OF THE BIG QUESTIONS ARE:

- Is your diet providing enough of these vitamins and minerals to keep the biochemical reactions working optimally?

- Does your diet provide sufficient plant chemicals to protect you against damage and disease?

- Are you in that unenviable place where you find out too late that a deficiency of certain micronutrients over time may have played a part in a particular health condition developing and pharmaceutical drugs now look like the only answer?

- Have you been struggling to lose weight for some time and wonder if perhaps nutrient deficiencies may be involved?

DOES ANYONE HAVE THE ANSWERS TO ANY OF THESE QUESTIONS?

Yes and No! What is becoming increasingly evident is that a diet based around highly processed, fast and junk foods, providing little in the way of fresh, nutrient-rich produce is regarded as a diet that not only increases our risk of malnutrition (ie provides less than adequate levels of vital nutrients) but also may increase our risk of disease.

What we don't know is whether, even though we may be focusing 24/7 on our diet and doing everything we can to get as much goodness into our day as we possibly can, we may still run short on certain vitamins and minerals from time to time.

This is largely down to our 21st century lifestyles. Many of us work way too long hours, many of us wear stress like an extra jacket, many of us don't get enough sleep, many of us have money worries, many of us have difficult relationships, many of us have sick or elderly relations that demand a great deal of our time and many of us party till we drop when we get a bit of 'down time' and every single one of these scenarios makes demands on the body and uses up nutrients at a pace which often leaves us feeling fatigued both emotionally and physically.

Based on the physiological evidence confirming the fundamental role of vitamins and minerals in the metabolism of energy, I support the belief that deficiency may compromise the sequence of biochemical reactions necessary for transforming food into usable energy. I also support the view that because a great many of us are regularly faced with emotional or physical or environmental or physiological stress (or all 4) and when the body is under any kind of stress, not only are certain micronutrients required in order to manage what is taking place, biochemically within the body but others are depleted fairly quickly during the process, this results in a greater need for certain vitamins, minerals and accessory nutrients.

The debate rages on and research continues with regard to whether we should supplement our diet or not. However, whatever side of the fence you are on, there are a few reasonably clear indications of possible ongoing deficiencies which may help you to decide whether you may wish to consider any of my recommendations.

ALWAYS KEEP IN MIND THAT SUPPLEMENTS ARE ONLY EVER 'SUPPLEMENTARY TO A GOOD DIET' AND SHOULD NEVER BE REGARDED AS A REPLACEMENT - DIET COMES FIRST EVERY TIME!

Head to the back of the book for lists of the most common symptoms of deficiency of certain vitamins and minerals plus a few extras which may provide a little 'food for thought' before you dive in.

Having digested what you have read, you may recognise a few (or many) symptoms from which you regularly suffer and determine that as you may be mildly or perhaps even majorly deficient in certain vitamins, minerals and accessory nutrients, it's time to get the credit card out and make some meaningful purchases in a bid to make a difference.

But before you do, keep in mind that you are about to make some major changes to your diet and lifestyle and some of the symptoms from which you currently suffer may ease or disappear in the foreseeable future so don't go leaping into the unknown just yet!

The first thing I want to make very clear is that I do not advise self-diagnosis - if your symptoms give a strong indication that you may be deficient in one particular vitamin or mineral or maybe more, it is not advisable to simply start taking a specific supplement that targets that possible deficiency. Some micronutrients work cohesively together and others don't which is why the very best nutritional supplement companies spend a great deal of time and money on research before producing carefully balanced products.

IMPORTANT!

Should you be suffering from continued ill-health and be particularly concerned about possible and perhaps specific deficiencies, I strongly advise that you consult a fully-qualified and recognised nutritional therapist who will gather a great deal of information about your family health history, your current health, your diet and lifestyle and any possible intolerances before determining whether supplementation is required and if so, design a programme tailored to your needs.

What Do I Recommend?

MAJOR PLAYERS...

A Multivitamin and Mineral Combination: if you are in relatively good health, are following my diet recommendations but want to ensure that you are getting a comprehensive range of the important vitamins, minerals and accessory nutrients on a daily basis.

Omega 3 Fatty Acids: even for the most devoted oily fish and seed eaters, it can be hard to reach the levels of omega 3 fats now regarded as optimal for brain, heart, nerve, bone and immune health.

An Antioxidant Combination: in a bid to protect ourselves against cellular damage caused by the many stressors we are faced with daily, we need to really focus on ensuring that we have maximum protection but it's a big ask so I favour a supplemental boost.

Vitamin D: unless your life involves a good daily dose of sunshine and you regularly consume the foods that offer respectable levels (oily fish, eggs, mushrooms and milks), there is every chance that you may become deficient over time so a supplement should be considered.

ADDITIONAL PLAYERS...

Magnesium: a deficiency of this mineral is not unusual. Firstly because of diets which are insufficiently-rich in green leafy vegetables, nuts and seeds and legumes but also because stressful lifestyles use up our magnesium stores at a rather alarming rate. Furthermore, and perhaps of equal interest to those who are looking to 'change the way they shift fat forever' is that this mineral is fundamentally involved in blood sugar management. Good to optimum levels have been shown to prevent elevated glucose and insulin levels which may result in us craving sugary and starchy foods on a more regular basis and predispose us to type 2 diabetes.

Chromium: there is extensive data supporting chromium's ability to lower blood sugar levels and increase insulin sensitivity plus there is some very encouraging evidence that dieters manage cravings a great deal more successfully when supplementing chromium.

Curcumin: early studies indicate that this active antioxidant ingredient in the spice, turmeric may play a role in reversing many of the inflammatory and metabolic problems associated with obesity by improving blood-sugar control.

SUGGESTED PRODUCTS

Whilst I have no affiliation with any particular supplement companies and don't in any way profit from promoting their products, I am recommending those that have never let me down and are produced/ distributed by companies that are extremely reliable, honest and professional. However, there are many others that may be more convenient for you to buy dependent on where you live.

My advice is always to buy the best you can afford as the cheaper versions are often 'lighter' on the main players and 'richer' on the cheaper ones so you may have to take more to achieve the same benefit ... or ... they may not be too well absorbed so you don't get the maximum from them.

It's a minefield which is not easy to navigate but feel free to contact me for advice on any products you are considering.

A quick search on the internet will take you to suppliers of all the following:

Multivitamins and Minerals
Biocare One a Day Plus
Solgar V2000
Solgar VM-Prime
Nutri Advanced Multi Essentials

Omega 3s
Nutri Eskimo Advanced EPA Fish Oil
Dr Mercola Antarctic Krill Oil

Antioxidants
Higher Nature Super Antioxidant Protection
Viridian Antioxidant Formula
Dr Mercola Astaxanthin

Vitamin D
Nutrishield High Strength Natural Vitamin D
Dr Mercola Sunshine Mist Vitamin D
Biocare Liquid BioMulsion D
Pharma Nord Bio-Vitamin D3

Magnesium
Floradix Liquid Magnesium
Biocare BioMagnesium
Natural Vitality Natural Calm Magnesium Powder

Chromium
Life Extension Optimised Chromium
Higher Nature Chromium 200
Biocare Liquid Chromium
Biocare Sucroguard

Curcumin
Life Extension Super Bio Curcumin
Natural Factors Theracurmin

There are also many **daily packs** now available which offer multi-nutrient protection which some find more convenient:

Nutrishield Essentials and Premium
Biotech USA Daily Pack
Higher Nature Advanced Daily Support

VERY IMPORTANT!

Always consult your doctor or health practitioner before starting a supplement programme if you have an ongoing health condition, are on regular medication, are pregnant or breastfeeding or are under age 16.

FAST LANE DIET PLAN

Keeping it Simple!

I totally appreciate and acknowledge that there are a few very important things that I must always consider when I encourage people to embark on a new diet/fat loss plan:

To keep it as simple and straightforward as possible! Few of us can happily launch into a new programme if there are too many rules, endless instructions and each day finds us having to spend time we probably don't have continually referring to a diet plan.

To give dieters plenty of choice. Some of us may love fish or like nothing better than creating smoothies with immense enthusiasm every day but there's no 'one shoe size fits all' when it comes to the foods we like, the crazy demands of our busy lives or the kitchen time we have so choice is paramount if we are to 'stick with the programme'.

To encourage dieters to experiment. If we are to shift fat in record time and keep shifting fat until we reach our goal (and maintain a healthy weight thereafter and forever), there are likely going to be foods and drinks and lifestyle habits that my readers may be unfamiliar with but can make a meaningful difference so it would be selfish of me not to encourage them to 'give them a go'!

To offer alternatives. We all have our likes and dislikes and sadly, the incidence of food intolerances are on the rise so should you find that certain meal and snack recommendations are not going to work for you, please contact me though my website or through social media and I will be happy to suggest alternatives.

So… here is your 2 week diet plan which is simple and straightforward, offers plenty of choice, encourages a bit of experimentation here and there and because I am nothing short of an obsessive when it comes to exhaustively-testing every bite I recommend, ensures that every day in your diet is satisfying, bursting with nutritional goodness and downright delicious!

IMPORTANT!

Some like to follow a diet plan 'to the letter' and if that's you, I suggest you follow the recommended diet choices for **Days 1 to 6, Days 7 to**

11 and **Days 12 to 14** and should you decide to factor in **Soup and Juice Days,** do so on days 4, 8 and 12 or days 5, 9 and 13.

Alternatively, should you prefer to reduce the number of meal and snack choices you make for convenience or to ensure that you are ahead of the game to save shopping, prepping and cooking time or simply because there are specific choices that appeal more than others, you can **create your own diet plan** and repeat your preferred first meal of the day, lunch, evening meal and snack choices throughout the 2 weeks and be confident that your diet won't let you down.

Just be sure that diet boredom doesn't creep in however - that's the rock on which many dieters flounder!

All recipes involved in the diet can be found in your *Fast Lane Recipes*.

FIRST THING EVERY MORNING

- **whenever possible**, exercise for 30 to 45 minutes first thing in the morning (preferably outdoors)

- **optional** - have a small, dark, rich cup of freshly-made coffee (no milk or sugar) before you head out

- drink a large glass of still water when you return

- have a mug of hot lemon and ginger or a glass of cleansing juice (see recipes for both) while you get showered and dressed whether you have had time to exercise or not

FIRST MEAL OF THE DAY CHOICES

Breakfast time or early morning - **don't force breakfast down if you are not hungry, just have your first meal when you are.**

- scrambled eggs on toast
- overnight muesli
- creamy porridge with honey
- ham, eggs and tomato
- fresh fruit salad with crunchy yoghurt

- stuffed avocado
- breakfast bruschetta
- smoked salmon on rye
- breakfast frittata
- cottage cheese with fruit and vegetables

LUNCH CHOICES

- soup plus salad
- crisp breads plus smoothie
- warm salad plus juice
- pulse/grain bowl plus dressing
- lettuce wraps plus nuts/seeds
- sushi/sashimi plus soup cups or mugs

EVENING MEAL CHOICES

- meal in a bowl soups
- one pot wonders
- meal in a bowl salads
- very quick dinners
- curries and casseroles
- filling egg dishes

MID MORNING/MID AFTERNOON SNACK CHOICES *(optional)*

- hummus and raw vegetable sticks
- mixed olives with feta cheese
- fresh tomato juice with fresh nuts
- a cold boiled egg
- celery sticks with nut butter
- oatcakes or rice cakes topped with nut butter, mashed avocado or tzatziki and smoked salmon
- natural yoghurt with fresh fruit and nuts
- Vegetable discs with hummus, nut butter or soft goats cheese
- natural cottage cheese with fresh fruit and crushed nuts
- protein/energy balls
- avocado filled with tinned tuna and natural yoghurt
- nut-stuffed dates
- miso soup
- hard cheese with green grapes
- sprouted grains or beans

BEDTIME/BEDSIDE SNACK CHOICES *(optional)*

- oatcakes with cold, cooked turkey
- natural yoghurt with runny honey
- banana on its own or mashed onto a rice cake
- fresh cherries and/or a glass of Morello cherry juice
- scrambled egg on a rye cracker
- creamy porridge
- essential smoothie

DRINKS CHOICES

- Still and Sparkling Water with added fresh fruits, vegetables and/or herbs
- Coconut Water (great with ice, lime and coconut flakes)
- Teas (black, white, red, green, fruit, herb, matcha, chai) - no sugar
- Fresh Fruit Juices (always with a little protein)
- Fresh Vegetable Juices (watch the salt content)
- Coffee made with fresh beans (no sugar but perhaps a dash of cream!)
- Milks (dairy and non-dairy)
- *Switchel* (a reviving combination of ginger, apple cider vinegar, maple syrup, lemon juice and still or sparkling water - *see recipe*)

All recipes involved in your diet are in bold italics and can be found in your Fast Lane Recipes.

Diet Days 1 to 6

Your First Thing in the Morning Routine *(whenever possible)*

Breakfast/Early Morning
(choose one)

- ***Scrambled Eggs on Toast***
- ***Mixed Fruit with Crunchy Yoghurt***
- ***Stuffed Avocado***

Lunch
(choose one)

- ***Quinoa Vegetable Bowl with Thai Dressing***
- ***Light Chicken Broth plus Tomato, Basil and Feta Salad***
- ***Fabulous Warm Salad plus Super-Green Juice***

Evening Meal
(choose one)

- ***One Pot Chicken, Fish or Chickpeas***
- ***Very Quick Salmon, Lamb or Tofu***
- ***Aubergine Curry***

If you exercise strenuously later in the day before your evening meal you may wish to add some unrefined starch to satisfy hunger and replenish muscle glycogen levels (optional)

- 2 tablespoons cooked grains (amaranth, barley, buckwheat, bulgur, farro, freekeh, kamut, millet, quinoa, brown rice, wild rice, spelt, teff)
- 2 tablespoons cooked beans or lentils
- 1 medium-sized sweet potato, baked or 'chipped' and oven-roasted
- 1 slice sprouted seed bread

Mid Morning and/or Mid Afternoon Snacks
(optional - choose one or two)

- a small pot of hummus with a selection of raw vegetable sticks
- a small bowl of mixed olives with feta cheese
- a glass of fresh tomato juice with a handful of fresh, mixed nuts
- 2 rice cakes topped with nut butter or mashed avocado
- 2 slices of hard cheese with a handful of green grapes
- a small carton of natural cottage cheese mixed with diced fresh fruit and crushed nuts
- 2 thick discs of cucumber, tomato, radish, courgette or apple topped with hummus, nut butter or soft goats cheese

Bedtime or Bedside Snack
(optional - choose one)

- 2 oatcakes with 2 slices of cold, cooked turkey
- a small carton of natural yoghurt with one teaspoon runny honey
- half a banana
- a handful of fresh cherries

Drinks Throughout the Day
*(between meals rather than with meals - choose from your **Drinks Choices** and remember to have a glass of water before every meal and snack)*

Diet Days 7 to 11

Continue with your preferred day 1 to 6 choices or add some or all of the following:

Your First Thing in the Morning Routine *(whenever possible)*

Breakfast/Early Morning
(choose one)

- *Breakfast Bruschetta*
- *Overnight Bircher Muesli*
- *Ham, Egg and Tomato*
- *Smoked Salmon on Rye*

Lunch
(choose one)

- *Lettuce Wraps plus Mixed Nut/Seed Mixes*
- *Soup plus Salad*
- *Crisp Breads plus Smoothie*

Evening Meal
(choose one)

- *Meal in a Bowl Soup*
- *Filling Egg Dish*
- *Very Quick Chicken, Burger or Prawns*
- *Singapore Noodles*

If you exercise strenuously later in the day before your evening meal you may wish to add some unrefined starch to satisfy hunger and replenish muscle glycogen levels (optional)

- 2 tablespoons cooked grains (amaranth, barley, buckwheat, bulgur, farro, freekeh, kamut, millet, quinoa, brown rice, wild rice, spelt, teff)
- 2 tablespoons cooked beans or lentils
- 1 medium-sized sweet potato, baked or 'chipped' and oven-roasted
- 1 slice sprouted seed bread

Mid Morning and/or Mid Afternoon Snacks *(optional - choose one or two from the selection in the* **Recipe Section***)*

Bedtime or Bedside Snack

(optional - choose one from the selection in the **Recipe Section***)*

Drinks Throughout the Day

(between meals rather than with meals - choose from your **Drinks Choices** *and remember to have a glass of water before every meal and snack)*

Diet Days 12 to 14 and Beyond

Continue with your preferred day 1 to 11 choices or add some or all of the following:

Your First Thing in the Morning Routine *(whenever possible)*

Breakfast/Early Morning
(choose one)

- *Creamy Porridge*
- *Breakfast Frittata*
- *Cottage Cheese with Fruits and Vegetables*

Lunch
(choose one)

- *Pulse/Grain Bowl plus Dressing*
- *Sushi/Sashimi plus Soup*
- *Warm Salad plus Juice*

Evening Meal
(choose one)

- *Meal in a Bowl Salad*
- *One Pot Wonder*
- *Curries or Casserole*

If you exercise strenuously later in the day before your evening meal you may wish to add some unrefined starch to satisfy hunger and replenish muscle glycogen levels *(optional)*

- 2 tablespoons cooked grains (amaranth, barley, buckwheat, bulgur, farro, freekeh, kamut, millet, quinoa, brown rice, wild rice, spelt, teff)
- 2 tablespoons cooked beans or lentils
- 1 medium-sized sweet potato, baked or 'chipped' and oven-roasted
- 1 slice sprouted seed bread

Mid Morning and/or Mid Afternoon Snacks *(optional)*
*(choose one or two from the selection in the **Recipe Section**)*

Bedtime or Bedside Snack
*(optional - choose one from the selection in the **Recipe Section**)*

Drinks Throughout the Day
*(between meals rather than with meals - choose from your **Drinks Choices** and remember to have a glass of water before every meal and snack)*

A 'Grab and Go' Day

Even with the very best intentions, it happens and suddenly you are faced with a day where you didn't plan ahead, there's little or no time to cook and you either have to depend on what is lurking in the fridge and/or whatever 'convenience' foods you can pick up during the day! Stick with the following advice and all will be well - just try not to let these days happen too often!

Generally, the best way to handle a 'grab and go' day is to snack regularly to keep your energy levels up when there's little time to sit down and savour the eating experience. However, regular snacking requires a bit of diligence if you don't want to 'undo the diet':

- every snack should be small
- as many snacks as possible should include some protein
- every snack should be light on starchy carbohydrates
- at least 2 snacks in your day should include fats

- have no more than 5 or 6 snacks in a day
- try to leave around 3 hours between each snack
- drink a glass of water before each snack
- have all other 'drinks choices' between snacks

Option 1: Grab some 'quick eats' from the fridge, cupboards, fruit bowl etc, sling them in a bag or box and dig in throughout the day. **Here's a selection of 'dependables':**

Hummus, natural cottage cheese, hard boiled eggs, fresh nuts and seeds, cheese portions, tinned fish, cold cooked meats, cooked prawns, leftover soup, cooked chicken portions, oatcakes/rye crackers/rice cakes, tomatoes, carrots, cucumber, celery stalks, avocado, olives, natural yoghurt, fresh fruit, no-sugar nut butter, no-sugar nut and seed bars, protein balls, goji berries, edamame beans, vegetable crisps.

Option 2: If the fridge and cupboards are relatively bare and you have to depend more on 'convenience' for the day, choose from the following snack combinations and remember to 'go small' with portion sizes:

- fruit smoothie plus a small pack of mixed nuts and seeds
- small carton of natural yoghurt plus a handful of berries or mixed fruit
- instant or ready-made porridge plus honey or spice topping
- **off the shelf soups**: go for those that are rich in vegetables plus beans, lentils, meat, poultry, fish, shellfish or tofu and avoid those that are creamy or with pasta, noodles, rice and other grains
- **off the shelf salads**: go for those that are rich in vegetables and salad leaves plus beans, lentils, rice, quinoa, meat poultry, fish, shellfish or tofu and avoid those with creamy dressings, pasta or noodles
- a small pot of hummus with a selection of raw vegetable sticks
- a small bowl of mixed olives with feta cheese
- a glass of fresh tomato or other vegetable juice with a handful of fresh, mixed seeds
- 2 rice cakes topped with nut butter or mashed avocado
- 2 oatcakes with sliced cold meat and/or chopped egg

- 2 seeded rye crackers with mashed banana
- **off the shelf protein shakes**: keep an eagle eye on the sugar content - many are not what they may seem!

If by chance you get time to sit down and eat and the choice is horribly limited to what looks like everything that is starch-rich and waistline-compromising either go for a breakfast-style option (eggs, bacon, tomatoes and mushrooms and steer clear of the toast) or a portion of meat/fish with vegetables or salad and steer clear of pasta, rice, potatoes, fries etc.

And if you are travelling and room service is your only option, don't open the mini bar other than to perhaps get some fruit or vegetable juice and still or sparkling water out and order an omelette or burger with no bun and no fries but lots of salad and/or vegetables or a protein-rich salad or soup of the day without rolls or bread.

WARNING!

If your day somehow or other miraculously calms down in the evening, don't be tempted to sit down to one of the recommended Evening Meals in your diet plan. This is a 'small and often snacking day' so stick with the suggestions.

A Soup and Juice Day

These are optional but should you choose to include them, I recommend days 4, 8 and 12 or days 5, 9 and 13

- **the evening before you start**: have your last meal of the day between 7pm and 8pm
- have a hot bath and go to bed early
- **first thing in the morning:** a mug of *Hot Lemon and Ginger*
- **around 10am**: a juice plus an only just ripe banana
- **around noon**: a generous bowl of soup
- **2pm to 3pm**: a cup or mug of soup
- **4pm to 5pm**: a juice plus an oatcake topped with hummus, cottage cheese or nut butter
- **7pm to 8pm**: a generous bowl of soup
- have a hot bath and go to bed early

SOUP CHOICES

- *Light Chicken or Lentil Broth*
- *Roasted Red Pepper and Tomato Soup*
- *Pea Mint and Lettuce Soup*
- *Blazing Hot Tomato Soup*
- *Spicy Turkey Soup*
- *Spinach and Watercress Soup*

JUICE/SMOOTHIE CHOICES

- *Essential Smoothie*
- *Very Berry Smoothie*
- *Apple, Pear and Lemon Smoothie*
- *Mango, Orange and Mint Smoothie*
- *Super-Green Juice*
- *Beta Carotene Cocktail*

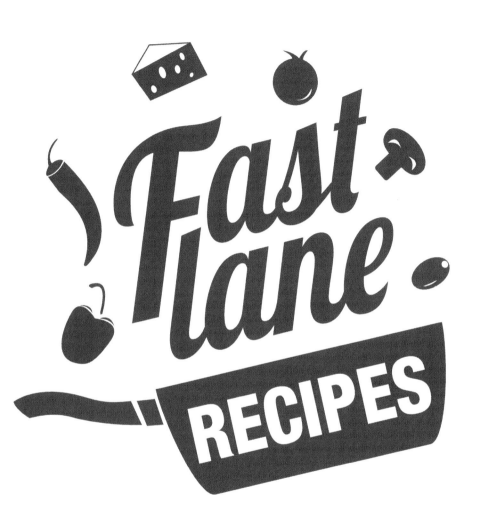

4

A Quick Word About My Recipes

I work with kilograms and grams for solids, litres and millilitres for liquids and tablespoons and teaspoons for ingredients that are required in smaller amounts - simply because it's the way I cook and always have! Should you be more used to cups, pounds, ounces, quarts and pints etc. I recommend you download one of the many super-quick and easy calculator apps. I use *Kitchen Calculator Pro* which rarely lets me down but there are lots out there so have a look around and find one that suits.

Wherever possible I use the very freshest ingredients available and make my own stocks for soups and stews but not every day goes to plan which is where a well-stocked cupboard and a freezer full of essentials is vital.

There are foods that merit different names in different parts of the world, there are also some that can be difficult to find dependent on where you live - but thanks to the internet, a quick search should keep you right and enable you to find the required item or a worthy alternative!

Some of my recipes make one serving for 'diet convenience' and others, particularly those that can be refrigerated or frozen in portions, serve 2 or 4. I heartily recommend you try to find some time whenever you can to get into the kitchen and prepare for the week ahead - you will feel justifiably smug if you do! However, should you have queries about doubling, halving or quartering any recipes, don't hesitate to contact me.

First Meal of the Day Choices

Scrambled Eggs on Toast

(makes 1 serving)

INGREDIENTS

- 2 large eggs
- Sea salt and freshly ground black pepper
- 1 thick or 2 thin slices sprouted seed bread
- Top quality butter

EXTRAS:

- smoked salmon offcuts, diced ham, grated hard cheese, chives, herbs

METHOD

Have your bread ready in the toaster or ready to go under a hot grill.

Put a small non-stick pan over a medium heat.

Lightly beat the eggs in a bowl, season with salt and pepper, pour into the pan and start stirring gently (use a wooden spoon with a pointed end or a spatula to get to the very edges of the pan).

Keep scrambling until three-quarters of the egg is a creamy mass then turn off the heat.

Toast the bread while you add 'extras' to the egg, if using and keep stirring until there is no liquid egg left.

Quickly butter your toast, top with the scrambled egg and dig in.

~

Why anyone would have a bowl of shop-bought cereal of a morning when you can have delectably-creamy scrambled eggs on hot buttered toast beats me!

Overnight Muesli

(makes 1 generous serving)

INGREDIENTS

- 6 tablespoons oats
- 140ml coconut water
- 2 tablespoons flaked almonds (toasted or un-toasted)
- ½ tablespoon Manuka honey
- 1 tablespoon full fat Greek yoghurt
- 2 teaspoons lemon/lime juice
- ½ apple, peeled, cored and grated
- 4 fresh mint leaves, very finely chopped

METHOD

Combine all the ingredients in a bowl, mix really well, cover and place in the fridge overnight. Serve with a sprinkling of cinnamon powder or grated nutmeg on top.

~

I learned how to make real authentic Bircher muesli whilst working as a waitress in the mountains of Switzerland in my early 20s. Since then, I have been playing around with the revered Dr Maximilian Bircher-Benner's classic, restorative recipe and this is one that doesn't include much fruit but still has a wonderfully sweet edge. The big bonus is that you can make it the night before and simply dive into the fridge in the morning for a helping or take it to work!

Creamy Porridge with Honey

(makes 2 servings)

INGREDIENTS

- 1 teacup medium-cut oats
- 3 teacups hot but not boiling water
- Decent pinch of salt
- Double cream
- Runny honey
- Cinnamon or nutmeg

METHOD

Place the water in a heat-proof bowl and gradually but meaningfully whisk in the oats - you don't want any lumps.

Leave to cool a little then cover the bowl and place in the refrigerator overnight.

In the morning (or whenever), transfer the porridge to a non-stick pan and cook over a medium heat until bubbling, stirring all the time.

Add the salt and continue to stir for another few minutes - if it is a little thick for your liking, just add some boiling water.

Serve with a spoonful or two of double cream, a drizzle of runny honey and a good sprinkling of cinnamon powder or grated nutmeg.

~

The fabulous thing about porridge is that there is no definitive recipe or cooking method - it's more of a personal thing. I am a Scot and over the years have sampled many a bowl of porridge - here's one of my fat-busting favourites where you soak the oats overnight so it takes less time to cook, is quickly ready to scoff or can be transported in a wide-necked vacuum flask.

Ham, Egg and Tomato

(makes 1 serving)

INGREDIENTS

- ½ tablespoon coconut or olive oil (or a mix of both)
- 2 medium free range eggs
- 2 thin slices Parma or other 'cured' ham
- 1 medium fresh tomato, halved
- Freshly ground black pepper

METHOD

In a small to medium-sized sauté pan, heat the oil over a medium heat until hot then add the tomato halves, flesh side down and cook for a few minutes then push them to the side of the pan.

Add the cured ham slices, let them sizzle for a minute or two before moving them to the side and cracking the eggs into the remaining space (turn the heat down if they start spluttering).

As the eggs cook, keep basting them with the oil using a spoon and tilting the pan slightly.

Once the eggs are cooked to your liking, season the eggs and tomato lightly with pepper (you are unlikely to need salt as the ham is 'salty') then lift all the ingredients onto a warmed plate with a slotted spoon or fish slice and dig in.

~

Once upon a time 'bacon and eggs' was regarded as a health-disrupting, only-on-a-Sunday breakfast treat but happily, no more..... have this quick and easy combo first thing in the morning or whenever.

Fresh Fruit Salad
with Crunchy Yoghurt

You can make your own 'crunchy mix' in bulk using grains, nuts and seeds of choice and store in a glass jar or other airtight container in the fridge or buy a ready-prepared muesli-type mix for convenience. If you go down that route, make sure it has no added sugars - label-reading is vital here and I recommend you head to a health store as a great many of those on the supermarket shelves are bulked out with dried fruits and involve difficult to spot sugary syrups!

INGREDIENTS

- Grains and flaked grains of choice (oats, millet, spelt, quinoa, buckwheat, rye etc)
- Nuts and seeds of choice
- Manuka honey
- Natural dairy or non-dairy yoghurt
- Fruits of choice
- Powdered cinnamon or grated nutmeg

METHOD

If you are making your own 'crunchy mix', preheat the oven to 150C/300F/Gas Mark 2-3.

Mix your chosen grains, nuts and seeds in a bowl, add a couple of tablespoons of runny honey and stir well until everything is coated.

Transfer the mix to a shallow baking tray and roast in the oven for 5 minutes. Remove from the oven, give the whole lot a good stir with a fork and return to the oven for another 5 minutes.

Remove from the oven and let the mix cool completely before transferring to an airtight container.

To serve, stir a couple of tablespoons of your homemade or ready-prepared 'crunchy mix' into 3 or 4 tablespoons of yoghurt, layer into a bowl or glass or transportable container with whole, sliced or diced fruit and top with powdered cinnamon or grated nutmeg.

~

The best thing about yoghurt, fruit and a bit of 'extra crunch' is that when you choose this as your first meal of the day, it is going to deliver an excellent balance of protein, fat and carbohydrate, make your taste buds sing and keep you firing on all cylinders until lunchtime!

Stuffed Avocado

I don't really do specific recipes for stuffed avocados - it's more a matter of what is in stock and how much time I can devote to creating and eating a tasty, filling and nutritionally-balanced, early morning combination.

Firstly: take a ripe avocado, half it, remove the stone, scoop the flesh out of both halves with a spoon and dice the flesh into a bowl with a good splash of lemon or lime juice to keep it from discolouring before deciding what to add.

If it's a large avocado, leave the stone in one half, paint the flesh with lemon/lime juice and wrap it tightly in cling film for later (or tomorrow). If it's a small avocado, use both halves.

Next: decide on what vegetables/fruit you want to add to the mix and dice, finely slice or grate them.

Then: add some protein and some sort of sauce or dressing and mix the whole lot into the diced avocado.

Finally: scoop your 'combination' into the empty avocado shells and top with some crunchy nuts and/or seeds.

Vegetable/Fruit Choices: tomatoes, cucumber, radishes, courgettes, carrots, peppers, chilli, roasted artichokes, olives, peas, corn, celery, spring onions, seaweeds, apple, pear, pomegranate, kiwi fruit, grapes, cherries.

Protein Choices: cold, cooked meats, cooked fish and shellfish, chopped egg, cooked beans, lentils and chickpeas, hummus, tofu, soft and hard cheeses.

Sauce/Dressing Choices: sour cream, mayonnaise, yoghurt, raita, salsa, extra virgin olive, avocado, nut and seed oils, horseradish, chutney, dressings.

Nuts and Seeds: fresh, roasted or toasted.

Here are a few of my favourite combinations:

Fresh prawns or crabmeat, sliced radish, chopped boiled egg, natural yoghurt and toasted pine nuts.

Tinned salmon, chopped boiled egg, sliced mixed olives, sliced cucumber, natural yoghurt, lemon juice and a good dash of smoked paprika powder.

Cottage cheese, grated courgette, grated apple, diced tomatoes, mango chutney and toasted flaked almonds.

Quickly sautéed bacon bits, sliced, ready-roasted peppers, raisins, parmesan shavings and shelled pistachios.

Breakfast Bruschetta

You can use whatever bread you like as long as it is open-textured. Go for the best you can find, slice it into nice thick ovals and keep them in the freezer for a speedy breakfast/first meal of the day.

Two other ingredients for a startlingly-good bruschetta are fresh garlic and a top quality cold-pressed peppery extra virgin olive oil. You may decide against the garlic at this time of the day (I don't but it's up to you).

METHOD

Toast a couple of slices of the bread under the grill on both sides until crispy around the edges and still ever-so-slighty spongy in the middle, wipe both sides with a peeled, halved clove of garlic, put them on a plate, drizzle the olive oil over - be generous - top with your chosen combo of goodies and devour.

SUGGESTIONS

Finely sliced fresh mozzarella, finely chopped ripe tomatoes, sea salt crystals, freshly ground black pepper and a couple of fresh basil leaves.

Thin slices of crisped up bacon or cured ham, sliced mushrooms sautéed in butter, scrambled egg and chopped chives.

Grated fresh courgette and apple or pear (use the biggest holes on a box grater), natural cottage cheese and lots of freshly ground black pepper.

Spread some fruity chutney from a jar over the base and follow with very thin slices of smoked ham and very finely sliced cucumber.

Nut butter, mashed fresh berries and watercress leaves.

Creamy goats cheese, baby spinach leaves, caramelised onions and crunchy, sliced radish.

Hummus, sliced avocado, grated raw carrot and toasted pine nuts.

Sliced banana, ricotta cheese and a good sprinkling of cinnamon powder.

Smoked Salmon on Rye

(makes 1 serving)

There are a number of reasons for the inclusion of this early morning meal. Apart from it being a deliciously filling way to start the day, it's hardly a chore to ensure there is smoked salmon in the fridge and dense, chewy, sliced rye bread in the fridge or freezer ready for toasting which makes the whole exercise super-quick. There are also lots of possible 'add-ons' for a bit of variety.

I favour pumpernickel which is hugely popular in Germany and Scandinavian countries for open sandwiches, comes ready-sliced and keeps in the fridge for up to a month.

Here are my '4 Ways' that require minimal preparation:

Have your bread ready in the toaster or ready to go under a hot grill - one slice is generally sufficient but if it's a very hungry morning, go for two and top with one of the following:

delicious creamy butter, sliced smoked salmon and lots of freshly ground black pepper

almond or cashew nut butter, sliced smoked salmon and finely-sliced cucumber

mashed or sliced avocado, sliced smoked salmon and finely-sliced peppery radish

horseradish sauce, sliced smoked salmon, chopped boiled egg and lots of freshly ground black pepper

~

I can also heartily recommend fresh, sliced pear and sliced/crumbled blue cheese or scrambled egg with chopped tomatoes or nut butter and sliced strawberries with a dash of Balsamic vinegar (it really works!)

Breakfast Frittatas

Quick, easy, filling and the variety of different frittatas you can make are only limited by your imagination!

As I am recommending them as a great first meal of the day, I accept that speed is of the essence so most of my suggested combinations require little preparation but you can part-make them the night before and pop them in the oven while you get showered and dressed.

A small, heavy-bottomed, oven-proof frying pan is a great and inexpensive investment for one-person frittatas.

I recommend 2 large or 3 small/medium free range eggs for a one-person frittata and enough filling to ensure that when 'the mix' goes into the pan, it is just visible above the egg rather than floating below the surface.

METHOD

Heat the oven to 160C/320F/Gas Mark 2–3.

In a large bowl, beat the eggs with a fork until lightly foamy and season with sea salt and freshly ground black pepper.

Prepare your fillings

Heat a little light olive, avocado or coconut oil in your pan over a medium heat and cook your fillings gently until cooked through (some like onions and peppers will require longer than those that are ready-cooked).

Once your filling is cooked through and looking tempting, pour the egg mixture into the pan and cook over a low heat for 3–4 minutes then transfer the pan to the middle shelf of the oven and cook for 6–8 minutes until the egg is set and golden on the surface.

GREAT COMBINATIONS:

- Ham, Courgette and Gruyere
- Smoked Salmon, Peas and Peppers
- Chicken, Spinach, Feta and Basil
- Bacon, Mushrooms, Cherry Tomatoes and Spinach
- Sautéed Onion, Fresh Chopped Herbs and Parmesan
- Smoked Trout, Crème Fraîche and Dill
- Spinach, Blue Cheese and Chives

~

If you are making your frittata the night before, stop the cooking after the 3-4 minutes in the pan on the hob, cover it and leave it in the fridge overnight and pop it in the oven for 6-8 minutes or until the egg is set on top the next morning

Cottage Cheese with Fruit and Vegetables

Over the years I have become accustomed to people telling me that try as they might, they simply don't like cottage cheese! However, this is never going to hold me back from recommending this low calorie, protein-rich, soft, mild-flavoured cheese that is packed with essential nutrients!

I think the slightly 'sour edge' is often the problem but this way of working it knocks that on the head so I urge you to give it a go. You can plate this, bowl it or box it to take to work or out and about early in the day.

Here's what you need for a one-person serving:

- 4 tablespoons natural cottage cheese
- 2 large, super-crispy lettuce leaves
- 2 tablespoons diced, cooked beetroot
- 4 cherry tomatoes, halved
- A good mix of whole, sliced or diced super-sweet fruits (berries, pineapple, pear, peach, nectarine, mango, papaya, passion fruit, melon, kiwi fruit etc)
- Sea salt and freshly ground black pepper (both are vital!)
- Balsamic vinegar (optional)
- A good handful of super-sweet, whole or chopped nuts (almonds, cashews, macadamias, pistachios etc)

METHOD

Pile the cottage cheese into the lettuce leaves and surround them with the beetroot, tomatoes and a selection of fruits.

Scatter a couple of good pinches of sea salt crystals, plenty of freshly ground black pepper and a drizzle of Balsamic vinegar over the lot (fruits included) then top with nuts.

SOUPS + SALADS

SOUPS

Pea, Mint and Lettuce Soup

(makes 4 bowls or 6 mugs)

INGREDIENTS

- 600ml frozen peas
- 600ml chicken or vegetable stock
- 1 old-fashioned round lettuce, cleaned and shredded
- A generous bunch fresh mint, chopped
- Sea salt and freshly ground black pepper
- 0% fat Greek yoghurt

METHOD

Put a couple of handfuls of the peas in a bowl, pour over some boiling water and leave to plump up while you make the soup.

Put the stock in a soup pot and bring to the boil.

Reduce the heat, add the rest of the peas and simmer until tender.

Turn off the heat and stir in the lettuce and mint.

Whizz in a blender or food processor until smooth (or the texture you prefer) then return to a clean pot and reheat gently.

Season to taste.

Ladle into bowls/mugs, top with a couple of teaspoons of yoghurt and quickly swirl with a skewer, drain the peas which have been soaking in the boiling water and scatter over before serving.

~

In this recipe, I use an old-fashioned round lettuce as it has that lovely sweet lettucey taste that is hard to beat but you can use all sorts and still get a great result (although I am not a fan of iceberg - tasteless!)

Spinach and Watercress Soup

(makes 4 bowls or 6 mugs)

INGREDIENTS

- 2 tablespoons light olive oil
- 1 medium onion, peeled and finely chopped
- 1 litre chicken or vegetable stock
- 1 heaped tablespoon porridge oats
- 300g spinach leaves
- 100g watercress
- Fresh lemon juice
- Sea salt and freshly ground black pepper

METHOD

Warm the oil in a large soup pot and sauté the onion gently until soft.

Add the stock and the porridge oats, bring slowly to the boil, turn down the heat and simmer for 15 minutes.

Add the spinach and watercress and keep stirring whilst bringing the soup back to the boil then turn off the heat.

Blend the whole lot until you have a smooth, foamy soup then return to a clean pan.

Heat through gently, add a good squeeze of lemon juice and check the seasoning.

You can grate a little lemon zest on top for added zing.

~

It is almost impossible not to start slurping this soup straight from the blender the minute you have blitzed it - the rich, green colour, the velvety smoothness and that subtle 'irony edge' that you just know is providing minerals in abundance makes this a quick-fix elixir you have to repeat again and again! And the oats add some protein making this a soup that fills you up for a good few hours...

Light Chicken or Lentil Broth

(makes 4 bowls)

INGREDIENTS

- 2 chicken thighs or 4 chicken wings or
- 4 tablespoons ready-cooked Puy lentils
- 1 tablespoon light olive oil
- 3 thick stalks celery, peeled and finely sliced
- 1 large onion, peeled and finely sliced
- 1 medium carrot, peeled and finely diced
- 1.2 litres chicken or vegetable stock
- 100g brown rice
- 1 teaspoon horseradish sauce
- A generous bunch of parsley, stalks removed and leaves very finely chopped
- Sea salt and freshly ground black pepper

METHOD

Roast the chicken pieces (if using) in a medium to hot oven until the skins are crisp and the flesh is cooked through while you make the soup.

Warm the oil in a soup pot, add the celery, onion and carrot and sauté gently until the vegetables are tender (about 15 minutes).

Add stock of choice and bring slowly to the boil.

Reduce the heat, add the rice and simmer very gently, covered until the rice is cooked (around 20 minutes).

Skin the chicken pieces and shred/chop the flesh before adding to the soup with the horseradish sauce and parsley or add the Puy lentils, horseradish sauce and parsley at this stage.

Stir well and season to taste.

As rice soaks up a lot of liquid, you will probably have to add more stock or water to achieve the light, brothy experience if you are not supping this soup immediately or have refrigerated/frozen it for future use.

NB: If you opt for the lentils instead of the chicken, you may wish to 'add a bit more green' in the form of shredded spinach or lettuce leaves or fresh/frozen peas towards the end of cooking.

~

This is a great broth to make in bulk and freeze in portions so you always have it on hand when you need a quick and nourishing lunch - it's good for much more than just the soul!

Gazpacho-Style Soup

(makes 4 bowls or 6 mugs)

INGREDIENTS

- 6 medium-sized, ripe tomatoes
- 1 large fennel bulb, trimmed, central stem removed and finely sliced/diced
- 450ml water
- 1 teaspoon sea salt
- 1 teaspoon coriander seeds
- ½ teaspoon black peppercorns
- 1 tablespoon light olive oil
- 1 small onion, peeled and finely chopped
- 1 large clove garlic, peeled and crushed
- ½ tablespoon Balsamic vinegar
- 1 tablespoon lemon juice
- 2 heaped teaspoons fresh oregano leaves, finely chopped
- 1 heaped teaspoon tomato purée
- Celery salt

METHOD

Put the tomatoes in a large bowl, cover with boiling water, leave for 30 seconds then drain and allow to cool a little.

Skin the tomatoes, quarter, remove the stems and seeds and chop the flesh roughly.

Put the fennel slices and water in a pot with the salt, bring slowly to the boil, turn down the heat, cover and simmer very gently for 10-15 minutes or until the fennel is tender but still has a bite to it.

Remove from the heat and set aside.

Crush the coriander seeds and peppercorns in a pestle and mortar or spice grinder.

Warm the oil in a soup pot, add the onion and ground spices and sauté gently until the onions are soft (don't let them brown).

Add the crushed garlic and sauté for a further 5 minutes.

Add the Balsamic vinegar, lemon juice, tomatoes, oregano leaves (leaving a few for topping the soup) and tomato purée and stir well.

Add the fennel with its simmering water, bring the soup to the boil then turn down the heat and simmer gently for 30 minutes.

Remove from the heat and let the soup cool a little before serving with a good shake of celery salt and a few chopped oregano leaves scattered over.

~

The 'hint of Spain' in this soup transports you to lazy days on holiday - this is the 'warm' version but it is also great served super-chilled in glasses...

Thai Prawn Noodle Soup

(makes 4 bowls)

INGREDIENTS

- 2 red chillies, de-seeded and roughly chopped
- 6 shallots, peeled and roughly chopped
- 3 cloves garlic, peeled
- 5cm piece fresh ginger, peeled and roughly chopped
- 1 stalk lemon grass, trimmed, bashed and sliced

- 1 teaspoon ground turmeric
- 1 teaspoon ground coriander
- 10g fresh parsley or coriander leaves
- 2 tablespoons coconut or light olive oil
- 2 x 400ml tins coconut milk
- 400ml fresh fish stock
- 2 tablespoons fish sauce (nam pla)
- 2 x 220g bags frozen raw king prawns
- 150g thin cooked rice noodles (optional)
- Sea salt and white pepper
- Juice of half a lime

METHOD

Blitz the chillies, shallots, garlic, ginger, lemongrass, ground turmeric, ground coriander, fresh parsley/coriander and oil in a food processor or spice grinder until you have a smooth paste.

Transfer to a soup pot and cook over a very gentle heat for 5 minutes.

Add the coconut milk and stock, bring just to the boil, quickly reduce the heat to very low and simmer for 10 minutes.

Add the fish sauce and prawns and simmer, stirring for a further 5 minutes until the prawns are bright pink.

Add the noodles (if using) and slowly bring back to just boiling.

Turn off the heat, season to taste, add the lime juice and let the soup stand for a couple of minutes before serving.

~

The secret to the success of this soup lies in the delicious paste that is very quick to prepare and emits a fragrance that invades the kitchen and prompts interest and enthusiasm from anyone passing through!

Parsley Soup with Chicken Nuggets

(makes 4 bowls or 6 mugs)

INGREDIENTS

- 2 tablespoons light olive oil
- 1 small onion, peeled and finely sliced/chopped
- 1 small courgette, cleaned and diced
- 1 x 28g pack parsley, washed, stalks separated and leaves roughly shredded
- 1 small clove garlic, peeled and sliced/crushed
- 400ml chicken or vegetable stock
- 1 small bay leaf
- Sea salt and freshly ground black pepper
- 1 small skinless chicken breast, chopped into bite-sized nuggets

METHOD

Warm 1 tablespoon of the oil in a soup pot, add the onion and courgette and gently sauté until tender but not coloured.

Add the parsley stalks and garlic and continue to sauté for a further 5 minutes.

Add the stock and bay leaf, bring to the boil, reduce the heat and simmer until the onions and courgette are soft.

Add the parsley leaves, bring back just to the boil then remove the pot from the heat.

Remove the bay leaf then transfer the soup to a blender and blitz until very smooth.

If it is a little too thick for your liking, add more stock or boiling water.

Strain through a fine sieve into a clean pot, check the seasoning and keep on a low heat until ready to serve.

Put the remaining tablespoon of oil, a good pinch of salt and a few grindings of black pepper in a bowl, add the chicken 'nuggets' and stir until well-coated, transfer to a baking sheet lined with tinfoil and grill under a medium heat, turning regularly until slightly crisp on the outside but still juicy inside.

Drain on kitchen or greaseproof paper, ladle the soup into bowls or mugs and top generously with the nuggets.

~

This has become a great favourite with my soup fans... it is crazily-green, bursting with goodness and makes a great 'to go' soup if you flask it... you can also top it with other grilled meats, tofu croutons or toasted nuts and seeds for a bit of variety.

Silky-Smooth Celery Soup

(makes 4 bowls or 6 mugs)

INGREDIENTS

- 1 tablespoon light olive oil
- 1 tablespoon top quality butter
- 400g celery stalks, leaves removed then peeled and diced
- 1 medium-sized potato, peeled and diced
- 2 large leeks, white parts only, finely sliced then rinsed
- 1 teaspoon celery salt
- Good pinch ground white pepper
- 500ml chicken or vegetable stock
- 300ml full fat or semi-skimmed milk

METHOD

Warm the oil and melt the butter in a soup pot, add the celery, potato, leeks, celery salt and white pepper, stir well and sauté over a very low heat for 30 minutes or until the vegetables are cooked through and soft. Check and stir every now and then to ensure nothing is browning at the base of the pot.

Add the stock, stir well, bring just to the boil then turn down the heat and simmer gently for a further 10-15 minutes.

Turn off the heat, leave to cool for around 5-10 minutes then stir in the milk.

Transfer to a liquidiser or blender and blitz until the soup is very smooth and frothy before straining, through a fine sieve into a clean pot and reheating gently.

Check the seasoning, adding a little more celery salt and white pepper to taste before serving topped with crisply fried, finely sliced onions or mushrooms or chopped fresh celery/parsley leaves.

~

I have lost count of the number of people who tell me they hate celery but once they have risked a bowl - love this soup... it's so creamy and delicious!

Blazing Hot Tomato Soup

(makes 4 bowls or 6 mugs)

INGREDIENTS

- 1 tablespoon light olive oil
- 1 medium onion, peeled and finely chopped
- 1 clove garlic, peeled and crushed or finely sliced
- 1 x 400g tin chopped tomatoes or 8 good-sized, fresh, ripe tomatoes
- 1 teaspoon sea salt
- 120g sweet red peppers in oil from a jar
- 500ml good chicken or vegetable stock
- ¼ teaspoon cayenne pepper
- ¼ teaspoon ground cumin
- ¼ teaspoon dried oregano
- ¼ teaspoon smoked paprika powder
- Juice of 2 small limes
- Natural live/bio yoghurt

METHOD

Warm the oil in a heavy-based soup pot, add the onion, garlic and salt, cover and sauté over a very low heat for around 20-30 minutes (the longer the better). Check and stir every 5 minutes or so to ensure the vegetables are not catching on the bottom of the pot.

If you are using fresh tomatoes, place them in a large bowl, pour boiling water over to cover, count slowly to 30, drain off the water, leave the tomatoes until cool enough to handle then slip off the skins, remove the core and seeds and roughly chop the flesh.

Drain the red peppers, slice and add to the pot with the tinned or fresh tomatoes, stock and spices and stir well - if you like it a little less 'hot', leave out the cayenne pepper - then bring just to the boil before turning the heat down to low and simmering for 20 minutes.

Blitz the soup in a blender before passing through a fine sieve into a clean pot, add the lime juice a tablespoon at a time and keep tasting until you get the perfect 'citrus edge', add sea salt to taste, reheat gently and serve topped with a generous spoonful of yoghurt straight from the fridge and a sprinkling of smoked paprika powder.

~

This soup can be as 'blazingly hot' as you want it - some like it hotter than others! When you add less of the spices (eg: just a pinch of two of the cayenne and smoked paprika powders) it tastes remarkably like a rather famous canned soup but without the added colourings, flavourings and preservatives so can be a real winner on the health stakes for both kids and those who don't go in for an overly-spicy soup. Packs well too!

Spicy Turkey Soup

(makes 4 bowls or 6 mugs)

INGREDIENTS

- 1 tablespoon light olive oil
- 1 large clove garlic, peeled and crushed
- 1 red chilli, de-seeded and finely sliced
- 1 onion, peeled and finely chopped
- 1 bunch spring onion, cleaned and finely sliced
- Small pack of pancetta cubes or 75g lean bacon, cubed
- 1 teaspoon dried oregano
- Generous pinch cayenne pepper
- Generous pinch ground cumin
- Freshly ground black pepper
- 1 x 400g tin peeled chopped tomatoes
- 1 litre chicken or vegetable stock
- 1 bay leaf
- Good pinch sea salt
- 1 turkey drumstick, skin off or 2 chicken drumsticks, skin off
- 3 tablespoons frozen peas or mixed peas and corn
- 1 good handful fresh coriander or parsley leaves, chopped
- Fresh lime juice

METHOD

Warm the oil in a soup pot, add the garlic, chilli, onion and spring onions and sauté very gently for 10-15 minutes until the onions are soft and translucent (don't let them brown).

In a small non-stick frying pan, sauté the pancetta/bacon until it is just browned around the edges. Drain on kitchen paper before adding to the soup pot.

Add the oregano, cayenne pepper, ground cumin and a few grindings of black pepper and stir well.

Add the tomatoes, stock, bay leaf, salt and turkey/chicken drumsticks and bring slowly to the boil, quickly reduce the heat and simmer gently until the meat is cooked and falling off the bone (around 35-40 minutes).

Add the frozen peas or peas and corn and simmer for another 8-10 minutes.

Remove the bay leaf, transfer the drumstick or drumsticks to a board and shred the cooked meat with a couple of forks before returning to the pan for a couple of minutes.

Top with the chopped coriander/parsley and add a splash of fresh lime juice before serving.

~

You can play around with the spices in this soup and make it more or less herby, spicy, 'hot' or 'cool' and use smoked bacon to add a smokey note. You can also use frozen broad beans instead of or with the peas or peas and corn - experiment!

SALADS

Crab, Salmon, Avocado, Fennel and Apple Salad

(makes 4 servings)

INGREDIENTS

- Cider vinegar
- Water
- Sugar
- Sea salt
- 1 bulb fennel, trimmed, root removed and very finely sliced
- 150g fresh white crab meat, flaked
- 5 drops Tabasco
- Fresh lemon juice
- 2 avocados, skinned, stoned and roughly chopped
- 100g good quality (or homemade) mayonnaise
- 100g crème fraîche

- 30ml fresh lime juice
- 1 green apple, cored and diced
- 100g smoked salmon in thin slices
- Freshly ground black pepper

METHOD

Combine a teaspoon of salt, a teaspoon of sugar, 1 tablespoon cider vinegar and 1 tablespoon water in a small pot, bring just to the boil, turn off the heat, add the fennel, cover and set aside until cool.

Mix the crab meat with the Tabasco and a dash of lemon juice, grind in some black pepper, cover and set aside.

Mash the avocado with a fork (or in a blender) with the mayonnaise, crème fraîche and lime juice until it is smooth and creamy.

Place the smoked salmon slices on a serving plate, scatter the diced apple around, drain the pickled fennel and add to the plate along with the crab mix, drizzle the avocado 'cream' over the whole lot, scatter more freshly ground black pepper around and serve.

~

This is a particularly delightful mix and the addition of the pickled fennel and avocado 'cream' are (I have to say, modestly) inspired!

Tomato Basil and Feta Salad

(makes 1 serving)

METHOD

Slice 2 large tomatoes (best, freshest, ripest and sweetest you can find) and plate with 6-8 shredded basil leaves and lots of crumbled feta cheese. Scatter hemp hearts (if you haven't tried these, you are in for a treat - they are seriously moreish!) or toasted pumpkin seeds over the top, season and lightly dress with Balsamic vinegar and top quality cold-pressed extra virgin olive oil.

~

This salad is all about really-fresh and 'best you can find' ingredients but in the winter months when fresh tomatoes can be a bit of a hit and miss affair, I recommend you coat them in olive or avocado oil and roast them in a very low oven until they are slightly caramelised around the edges and become nicely sweet.

Smoked Trout and Lentil Salad

(makes 4 servings)

INGREDIENTS

- 125g ready-cooked Puy lentils
- 2 shallots, peeled and very, very finely chopped
- 2 tablespoons extra virgin olive oil
- 1 teaspoon sherry vinegar
- Sea salt and freshly ground black pepper
- 2 cloves garlic, peeled and crushed or grated
- 200g smoked trout, cut into long, thin ribbons
- Fresh coriander leaves, finely chopped

METHOD

In a medium-sized pot, combine the lentils, shallots, oil, vinegar, a good pinch of salt, lots of pepper and the garlic over a low heat until everything is nicely warmed through.

Plate the lentil mix (you can serve it warm or let it cool a little or even go cold - works every which way), arrange the smoked trout slices in twists and scatter plenty of coriander about.

~

This is a demon of a salad and ticks a whole load of health-enhancing boxes!

Omega Salad

(makes 2 servings)

INGREDIENTS

FOR SALAD:

- Mixed raw greens - spinach, kale, watercress, parsley and Brussels sprouts - all very finely sliced
- Lightly steamed broccoli and cauliflower florets
- Kidney beans (tinned are fine - rinse well)
- Omega 3-rich eggs - boiled, cooled, shelled and halved
- Cold, cooked mackerel, sardines, rainbow trout, prawns or crabmeat or Strips of grass-fed beef, lightly sautéed or Tofu, cubed, coated in olive oil and baked in the oven until crisp
- Mixed seeds (pumpkin, sunflower, hemp, sesame)
- Fresh walnut halves

FOR DRESSING:

- 2 tablespoons extra virgin olive oil
- 2 tablespoons unrefined flaxseed oil
- 1 tablespoon apple cider or white wine vinegar
- 1 teaspoon grainy or smooth mustard
- Drizzle of runny honey
- Sea salt and black pepper to taste

METHOD

Sauté the beef (if using).

Bake the tofu (if using).

Steam the broccoli and cauliflower florets.

Boil the eggs.

Prepare the dressing.

Pile everything except the dressing into a bowl or container.

Keep the dressing separate and mix in just before serving (don't drench the salad).

~

A good daily dose of Omega 3 fatty acids are crucial for a sharp brain and a lean and healthy body and a mixed lunchbox salad is a great way of getting a load of them into your busy life. Experiment and create your own tasty and portable combinations.

Energy Salad

(makes 1 serving)

INGREDIENTS

FOR SALAD:

- Mixed salad leaves
- Steamed green beans and broad beans (shell these before adding)
- Spring onions, very finely sliced
- Grated raw courgette/zucchini (wiped but not peeled)
- Grated apple (wiped but not peeled)
- Beansprouts
- Cold, cooked chicken, turkey, duck or venison, finely sliced and/ or Cooked, drained and rinsed chickpeas (try and get the ones that come in jars - they are always tastier than the ones in tins)
- Natural cottage cheese
- Toasted flaked almonds

FOR DRESSING:

- 2 tablespoons white wine vinegar
- 1 tablespoon rice wine vinegar
- 1 teaspoon soy sauce
- ½ garlic clove, peeled and minced
- ½ inch piece fresh ginger root, peeled and minced

- 1 teaspoon sesame oil
- 4 tablespoons avocado oil

METHOD

Steam the green beans and broad beans and leave to cool a little.

Prepare the dressing by mixing everything in a jar or whisking in a bowl.

Pile everything except the dressing into a container.

Keep the dressing separate and mix in just before serving (don't drench the salad).

~

You can really play around with this salad, adding more or different lightly-steamed greens if you wish, substituting whatever proteins you have in stock and adding toasted mixed nuts and seeds in place of the flaked almonds. You can also opt for a different dressing - but I wouldn't recommend it as this one is a real winner!

Lentil and Bean Salad

(makes 4 servings)

INGREDIENTS

- 230g ready-cooked Puy lentils
- 230g tinned kidney beans, drained and rinsed
- 80g natural cottage cheese
- 80g raisins
- 40g dried apricots, chopped
- 40g cashew nuts, chopped
- 2 tablespoons top quality mayonnaise
- 2 tablespoons natural live/bio yoghurt
- Lemon juice to taste
- Sea salt and freshly ground black pepper
- Watercress

METHOD

Gently mix all the ingredients together and chill before serving with the watercress.

~

I'm not sure whether it is the cottage cheese/mayo/yoghurt mix that adds a 'killer' extra dimension or the addition of the chopped nuts but whatever it is, it works really well and because it can live happily for a couple of days in the fridge, makes a seriously good and easily-transported lunch when your day is full-on. And of course, you can play around with it and use different beans, lentils, dried fruits and nuts and seeds!

Green Salad with Loads of Extras!

A mixed, dressed green salad is a great accompaniment to lunch or dinner but it's all too easy for it to be slightly dull! Here are a selection of ideas that will make it sing!

Leaves: start with a mix of crunchy, soft and delicate, peppery and sweet - rocket, cos, romaine, lambs lettuce, round, oak leaf, chard, endive, escarole, mazuna, spinach, watercress, mustard cress, herbs, beet greens

Dressing: keep it simple with just a good quality cold-pressed extra virgin olive, avocado or cold-pressed extra virgin rapeseed oil and a dash of fresh lemon or lime juice or go for one of my suggested dressings.

Extras: staying with the 'green theme' you can add very finely-sliced cabbage, Brussels sprouts, kale, spring onions, beansprouts, grated or diced courgette, blanched or steamed green beans, broad beans, peas, broccoli florets, asparagus, bok choy or samphire and... add a few green, shelled pistachios for extra crunch!

The most important thing here is to ensure that everything that goes into the salad is super-fresh and if you are transporting it for later, keep the dressing separate and mix it through (with your hands is best!) just before you get stuck in.

CRISP BREADS

Select plain wholegrain rye crisp breads or the ones with added grains and/or mixed seeds and top with one of the following delicious combinations or simply get creative and become a crisp bread guru!

Sliced cooked beef, tzatziki, toasted flaked almonds, fresh mint leaves and a drizzle of honey.

Fresh prawns or crabmeat, sliced cucumber, chopped boiled egg, natural yoghurt and toasted pine nuts.

Parma ham, sliced raw mushrooms, sliced tomato, scrambled egg or sliced boiled egg and a dash of Worcestershire sauce.

Tinned tuna, coarse grain mustard, lime/lemon juice, anchovy sauce, sliced tomato and Greek yoghurt.

Tinned salmon, chopped boiled egg, sliced mixed olives, sliced avocado, sliced cucumber, natural yoghurt, lemon juice and a good dash of smoked paprika powder.

Smashed avocado, cottage cheese, grated courgette, cherry tomatoes and chutney.

Smoked salmon, raita, a dollop of horseradish sauce, watercress and sliced apple.

Nut butter, mashed fresh berries and watercress leaves.

Creamy goats cheese, baby spinach leaves, caramelised onions and crunchy, sliced radish.

Hummus, sliced avocado, grated raw carrot and toasted pine nuts.

Sliced banana, ricotta cheese and a good sprinkling of cinnamon powder.

TOP TIP!

Remember to scribble down some of the combinations you come up with - it's all too easy to forget what works for you - build up a list of them so you can be sure you have your favourite ingredients in stock!

~

The great thing about crisp breads and toppings is that they are hugely convenient when you are busy and once you have decided on a few favourite toppings, it's not too onerous to throw a couple together at speed!

SMOOTHIES

Essential Smoothie

INGREDIENTS

- 2 tablespoons mixed raw seeds (pumpkin, sunflower, flax etc.)
- 100g watermelon, seeds included
- 200g mixed red/purple berries (raspberries, blueberries, blackcurrants, strawberries, stoned cherries, brambles etc.)
- 200g silken tofu, drained and sliced
- 750ml rice, oat, almond or soya milk

METHOD

Place the seeds in a spice grinder and blitz until pulverised or use a mortar and pestle.

Place 3 ice cubes in a blender with all the other ingredients and run on low power until they start to come together, then on full power until the smoothie is creamy and frothy.

Add a little water if it is too thick and strain to remove the seedy, gritty bits.

~

You can make more of the seed mix in one go and keep it in a dark glass jar in the refrigerator for up to a week for convenience.

Super Green Smoothie

INGREDIENTS

- 100g baby spinach leaves
- 100g romaine lettuce leaves
- 110ml chilled water
- 110ml unsweetened pineapple juice
- A good handful of frozen green grapes (bag and put them in the freezer the night before)
- ½ tablespoon protein powder, powdered greens or chia seeds (quickly grind the seeds in a spice grinder or with a pestle and mortar before adding)

METHOD

Place the spinach, lettuce and water in a blender and whizz until smooth. Add a few ice cubes if you haven't frozen the grapes.

Add the grapes and whizz again until smooth.

Add the pineapple juice and protein powder, powdered greens or ground chia seeds and give the whole lot a final whizz until smooth.

Very Berry Smoothie

INGREDIENTS

- 200g frozen mixed berries
- 110ml unsweetened pomegranate or apple juice
- 110ml water
- ½ tablespoon ground almonds
- ½ tablespoon flaxseed or coconut oil

METHOD

Combine all the ingredients in a blender and whizz until well-blended and very smooth and frothy.

Apple, Pear and Lemon Smoothie

INGREDIENTS

- 1 medium apple, cored and chopped
- 1 medium pear, cored and chopped
- 1 teaspoon peeled and grated fresh ginger
- 1 tablespoon oats
- Juice of half a lemon
- Coconut Water

METHOD

Combine all the ingredients in a blender and whizz until very smooth and frothy.

Use as much coconut water as you wish to reach your desired consistency.

Mango, Orange and Mint Smoothie

INGREDIENTS

- 1 large ripe mango, stoned, peeled and flesh diced
- 1 large or 2 medium oranges, peeled and chopped (make sure you remove any pips)
- 1 tablespoon fresh lime juice
- 4 fresh mint leaves, finely chopped
- 200ml natural yoghurt

METHOD

Place the mango, orange, lime juice, mint leaves and a teacup of very cold water in a blender and whizz until smooth.

Add the yoghurt and whizz again. If it is a little thick for your liking, add a little more cold water.

~

There are so many possible smoothie combinations! Just make sure you always add some protein - yoghurt, kefir, milks, cottage cheese, nuts and nut butters, seeds and seed butters, oats or protein powders.

WARM SALADS + JUICES

WARM SALADS

Fabulous Warm Salad

(makes 1 serving)

INGREDIENTS

- 1 tablespoon pine nuts
- 1 tablespoon olive or avocado oil
- ½ red pepper, de-seeded and finely sliced
- 4 spring onions, trimmed and finely sliced
- 1 skinless chicken breast, carved into bite-sized slices or smoked tofu, cubed
- Crunchy lettuce leaves, torn into edible bites
- ½ cucumber, peeled, seeds removed and thinly sliced
- ½ courgette, wiped and grated
- A handful of frozen peas, soaked in boiling water for 5-10 minutes
- A handful of beansprouts
- Large tomato, sliced or quartered
- ½ avocado, stoned, peeled and sliced

FOR THE DRESSING:

- 3 tablespoons extra virgin olive oil
- ½ tablespoon white wine vinegar or lemon juice
- 1 teaspoon coarse grain or Dijon mustard
- A pinch of sea salt
- Freshly ground black pepper

METHOD

Toast the pine nuts in a frying pan over a medium heat until golden and set aside.

Sauté the peppers and spring onions in the oil until soft and slightly caramelised around the edges then remove with a slotted spoon, cover and keep warm.

Add the chicken or tofu cubes to the remaining oil and sauté gently until cooked through and slightly crisp around the edges.

Meanwhile, mix all the dressing ingredients in a small pan or microwaveable dish and very gently heat through.

Load a good helping of the lettuce leaves into a wide serving bowl or transportable container, add the cucumber, grated courgette, peas and beansprouts then top the salad with the hot onions and peppers followed by the hot chicken or tofu and finally the tomato, avocado and pine nuts.

Drizzle the warm dressing over the whole dish but don't soak it, sit yourself down and enjoy!

This is just one suggested combination but you can really go to town with this type of salad using all different types of salad leaves, lightly sautéed meats, fish, shellfish and vegetables, cooked beans and lentils, finely sliced raw vegetables and fresh fruits, nut and seed mixes and various dressings. It's a perfect salad for using up whatever you have in stock.

NB: if you are transporting your salad, keep the dressing separate in a jam jar or secure container and warm it through at the last minute. You can also microwave the whole lot very briefly (30 secs tops). Everything wilts just a little but is rather delicious!

Beta Carotene Cocktail

INGREDIENTS

- 3 ice cubes
- 1 yellow or orange pepper, de-seeded and chopped
- 1 orange, peeled and chopped
- ½ small cantaloupe melon, peeled and chopped
- 4 fresh apricots, cleaned, stoned and chopped
- 4 cos lettuce leaves, washed and torn
- Fresh carrot juice

METHOD

Blitz the ice cubes, pepper, orange, melon, apricots and lettuce until smooth and add carrot juice until you achieve a juice consistency rather than a smoothie consistency.

Super Green Juice

INGREDIENTS

- 100g baby spinach leaves
- 100g romaine lettuce leaves
- 110ml chilled water
- 110ml unsweetened pineapple juice
- A good handful of green grapes

METHOD

Place the spinach, lettuce and water in a blender and whizz until smooth.

Add the grapes and whizz again until smooth.

Add the pineapple juice and give the whole lot a final whizz until smooth adding more chilled water if necessary to produce a juice consistency rather than a smoothie consistency.

Cherry and Apple Juice

INGREDIENTS

- 3 ice cubes
- 2 large handfuls of ripe cherries with stalks and stones removed (you can use tinned, stoned cherries in fruit juice - not syrup - and drain them for speed)
- 1 large tart apple, peeled, cored and chopped (a Granny Smith is good)
- Cold water

METHOD

Place the ice cubes, cherries and apple in a blender with a teacup of cold water, whizz until well-blended, then add more cold water until the whole thing is a sensational liquid concoction!

MORE DELICIOUS COMBINATIONS!

The secret to a good juice is not to keep piling in the ingredients assuming that the more there are, the greater the 'goodness' and the health benefits!

Many vegetables and fruits which complement each other on a plate don't always make such a great marriage in a juice.

Always start with a few ice cubes and some chilled water, always chop the vegetables and fruits into bite-sized chunks (and remove stones and pips where necessary) and always shred leaves and fresh herbs and the whole thing will come together fairly quickly. Also, always have some more chilled water to hand to achieve a juice rather than a smoothie consistency.

TRY SOME OF THESE:

- apple and blackcurrant
- blueberry, apple and lemon
- pink grapefruit, orange and pineapple
- tomato, celery, parsley and radish
- pear, melon and cucumber
- melon, apple and mint
- spinach, pomegranate, lime and basil
- pear, lime and tarragon
- peach, lettuce and strawberry
- mango and grapefruit
- papaya, passionfruit and grape
- orange, raspberry, ginger and dill

PULSE/GRAIN BOWLS + DRESSINGS

PULSE AND GRAIN BOWLS

Pulses and grains make a splendid base for both hot and cold one-bowl lunches and the selection available on the supermarket, deli and health store shelves is pretty mind-blowing!

Beans come in all colours, lentils too, then there are chickpeas and all manner of rice varieties before we even start getting our heads around 'ancient grains' like quinoa, farro, amaranth, barley, buckwheat, teff, freekeh etc!

You may already have a few favourites and if so, you may wish to stick with them for your lunch bowls but then again, you may be feeling adventurous and want to get a few new recruits into the kitchen cupboard!

The route to a good pulse and/or grain bowl (they work well together) is to start by cooking your pulses and grains (and cooling them if it's going to be a cold affair) but there are as many YouTube videos on how to 'cook them perfectly' as there are varieties so I have to confess I tend towards following the instructions on the packet!

Alternatively, if time is tight, you may decide to spend just a little more and buy the 'ready-cooked' or 'quick cook' tins or packs.

Next on the list is to add some sort of protein (meat, poultry, game, fish, shellfish, cheese, eggs, tofu - either hot or cold), then some finely sliced or diced lightly steamed or sautéed or raw vegetables (and perhaps some fresh or dried fruit), then some fresh, toasted or roasted nuts and seeds and finally, to bring the whole thing together to achieve a gloriously-colourful and deeply-delicious bowl of nutritional goodness, a dressing!

Here are a few of my favourites to get you started but I urge you to 'get creative' and with that in mind, I have included a selection of dressings which I promise will add something special to your efforts!

Quinoa Vegetable Bowl

(makes 2 bowls)

INGREDIENTS

- 50g quinoa, cooked according to package instructions
- 4 florets broccoli, finely chopped
- ½ small red onion, peeled and very finely diced
- 1 small carrot, scrubbed and roughly grated
- A handful of coriander leaves, roughly chopped
- 2 spring onions, very finely sliced
- 1 tablespoon fresh peanuts, chopped or roughly crushed

FOR THE DRESSING:

- Zest and juice of half a lime
- ½ teaspoon sesame seeds
- ½ tablespoon tamari

- ½ tablespoon sesame oil
- ½ tablespoon rice wine vinegar
- 1 clove garlic, peeled and minced/grated
- 2cm piece fresh ginger, peeled and minced/grated

METHOD

In a large bowl toss cooked quinoa, broccoli, red onion, carrot, coriander, spring onions and peanuts together. Mix until combined.

In a small bowl combine dressing ingredients.

Pour dressing over quinoa and mix until combined.

~

This is such a quick, tasty and protein-rich salad which you can happily mess around with dependent on your tastes and what's in stock. I have tried calves liver, shiitake mushrooms and blue cheese plus duck breast, dried cherries and mozzarella with good results - experiment!

Fennel and Orange Grain Bowl

(makes 2 bowls)

INGREDIENTS

- 100g quinoa, barley, amaranth, bulgur, faro, millet, spelt, teff, freekeh or brown rice
- 1 large or 2 small fennel bulbs, trimmed and divided into quarters or eighths (keep the root in place as this holds the segments together)
- 50ml fresh orange juice
- 1 pinch saffron powder
- Sea salt
- Freshly ground black pepper
- Light olive oil
- 1 tablespoon tahini paste

- 1 tablespoon flaked almonds
- 1 orange, skin and pith removed with a sharp knife and segmented
- 2 tablespoons pomegranate seeds
- 1 tablespoon finely chopped fresh chives
- Extra virgin olive oil

METHOD

Prepare the grains according to the cooking instructions.

Put the fennel in a bowl with the orange juice, saffron, a dash of salt and plenty of black pepper, cover and leave to 'infuse' for 20 minutes then drain (keeping the liquid), dry the fennel off with paper towel, lightly paint each quarter with the olive oil, place on a baking sheet under a hot grill and grill (turning often) until they are cooked through but still have a bit of 'bite' and are nicely caramelised.

Combine the tahini paste with the strained orange/saffron/fennel marinade until really smooth and creamy.

Toast the flaked almonds in a small dry frying pan - watch them like a hawk as they burn in the blink of an eye!

Fork through the grains until there are no clumps then mix the tahini dressing through before placing in a bowl or transportable container.

Arrange the grilled fennel and orange segments around, scatter the pomegranate seeds, chopped chives and almonds over the whole lot, drizzle some extra virgin olive oil over the salad and serve.

~

I love this salad on its own as it is so fresh, colourful and satisfying but it also makes a good 'side' to a thick fillet of baked 'meaty' fish like cod, halibut or turbot.

Creole Banana Rice Bowl

(makes 2 bowls)

INGREDIENTS

- 110g long grain rice
- 2 large bananas, peeled and sliced
- ½ tablespoon lemon juice
- ½ medium red eating apple, cored and chopped
- 50g seedless grapes
- 40g canned or fresh pineapple, chopped
- 1 tablespoon finely chopped walnuts or almonds
- ½ tablespoon sultanas
- Large lettuce leaves

FOR THE DRESSING:

- 3 tablespoons top quality bought or homemade mayonnaise
- 1 tablespoon lemon juice
- Good pinch hot chilli powder
- ¼ teaspoon dry English mustard

METHOD

Cook the rice according to packet instructions. Drain and allow to cool. Gently stir the bananas, lemon juice, apple, grapes, pineapple, walnuts or almonds and sultanas into the rice.

Mix together the mayonnaise, lemon juice, chilli powder and mustard and stir into the banana and rice mixture.

Arrange a few lettuce leaves in a bowl, pile the rice mixture on top, check seasoning and sprinkle over more chopped walnuts or almonds.

~

Sweet, sour, spicy and colourful. It also works well with kiwi, apricots, black grapes and pistachios in place of banana, pineapple, green grapes and walnuts/almonds.

Mixed Bean, Chicken and Chorizo Bowl

(makes 2 bowls)

INGREDIENTS

- 1 tablespoon light olive oil
- ½ red onion, finely chopped
- ½ red pepper, seeded and diced
- 50g chorizo, diced
- 1 small skinless chicken breast, finely sliced
- ½ teaspoon sweet paprika
- 1 heaped tablespoon corn kernels
- 1 heaped tablespoon tinned red kidney beans, rinsed
- 1 heaped tablespoon tinned cannellini beans, rinsed
- 1 heaped tablespoon pre-cooked brown rice
- 100g kale, hard stems removed and leaves finely sliced
- Sea salt and freshly ground black pepper
- Yoghurt dressing (see dressings)

METHOD

Heat the oil in a medium-sized pan over a medium heat. Add the onion and pepper and sauté gently until softened.

Add the chorizo and chicken and sauté until cooked through and slightly caramelised around the edges.

Add the paprika, corn, beans and rice, stir well and continue to cook until heated through.

Add the kale leaves and cook until just wilted, check the seasoning, transfer to a bowl, mix the dressing through and keep in an airtight container until ready to eat to let the flavours marry.

~

This is one of those 'bowls' you can really play around with. Try different beans, different 'greens', different meats or poultry and different dressings or keep it meat-free.

Mediterranean Chickpea Salad Bowl

(makes 1 bowl)

INGREDIENTS

- 2 tablespoons chickpeas, rinsed and drained
- 1 tablespoon red pepper, de-seeded and chopped
- 1 tablespoon yellow pepper, de-seeded and chopped
- 1 green bell pepper, chopped
- 1 tablespoon red onion, peeled and very finely sliced
- 6 cherry tomatoes, halved
- 2 teaspoons pitted black olives, halved
- 1 tablespoon diced cucumber
- 1 tablespoon feta cheese, crumbled
- Sea salt
- Freshly ground black pepper
- Italian Dressing (see dressings)

METHOD

Place all the ingredients in your bowl and mix well.

Add the dressing and check the seasoning.

Keep the dressing separate if you are transporting the salad to devour later.

NB: you can also add steamed green beans, broad beans, peas or asparagus and diced or sliced fresh peach gives this bowl a lovely fruity edge.

~

Summer on a plate! You can really go to town here, adding more colour, using different cheeses and other dressings!

DRESSINGS

You can prepare your dressings in a small bowl and whisk everything together until well blended then use immediately or store in an airtight container or use a jam jar with a lid and shake well, which is my preference.

If you are storing your dressing for later and it has been in the fridge, always let it come to room temperature and give it another good shake before use.

FRENCH DRESSING

Put a ¼ clove of peeled, crushed garlic, 1 teaspoon Dijon mustard, 2 tablespoons white wine vinegar (or half and half vinegar and lemon juice), 6 tablespoons extra virgin olive oil, a good pinch of sea salt and a few twists of freshly ground black pepper in a jar with a lid and shake well. Use immediately or store for up to 2 days.

ITALIAN DRESSING

In a small bowl, whisk together 1 tablespoon top quality or homemade mayonnaise, 1 tablespoon crème fraîche, 2 tablespoons extra virgin olive oil, 1 tablespoon red or white wine vinegar, ½ tablespoon grated fresh Parmesan cheese, 1 tablespoon fresh milk, ½ peeled and crushed garlic clove, 1 teaspoon very finely chopped fresh parsley, a pinch of sea salt and a few twists of black pepper and use immediately or store in the fridge for up to 2 days.

THAI-STYLE DRESSING

In a small bowl, whisk half a peeled and crushed garlic clove, 1 tablespoon soy sauce or tamari and 2 teaspoons rice wine vinegar. Whisk in 100ml avocado or light olive oil - gradually - then half a teaspoon sesame oil. Season with sea salt and freshly ground black pepper and use immediately or store in a cool place for up to 2 days.

LEMONY-ORANGE DRESSING

Combine one third of a peeled and very finely chopped shallot, 4 tablespoons extra virgin olive oil, 1 tablespoon white wine vinegar, 1 tablespoon fresh lemon juice, ½ tablespoon fresh orange juice and a teaspoon of grated lemon zest in a lidded jar and shake well. Season to taste with sea salt and freshly ground black pepper, shake again and use immediately or store in a cool place for up to 2 days (or keeps in the fridge for up to a week).

YOGHURT DRESSING

Put 5 tablespoons natural yoghurt, 2 tablespoons sherry vinegar, 1 tablespoon extra virgin olive oil, a pinch of smoked sweet paprika powder, a pinch of sea salt and a few twists of freshly ground black pepper in a lidded jar, shake well and use immediately or store in the fridge for no more than 1 day.

NUT BUTTER DRESSING

Place 1 heaped tablespoon coconut cream, 3 tablespoons boiling water, 3 tablespoons no-sugar nut butter (peanut, almond, cashew, macadamia, walnut etc), ½ teaspoon ground coriander, 1 peeled and finely chopped shallot, 1 tablespoon light soy sauce, ½ teaspoon peeled and finely grated fresh ginger, ½ de-seeded and finely chopped red chilli, a pinch of sea salt and a few grindings of black pepper in a small pan and over a gentle heat, stir until everything comes nicely together and the sauce is just beginning to bubble. Dress salad and/or bowls whilst still hot or leave to cool completely and store. You may need to add more water when cool.

LETTUCE WRAPS + NUT AND SEED MIXES

LETTUCE WRAPS

WRAP TIPS: Always use a tasty, crunchy lettuce (cos, romaine, little gem and raddichio are my choices) - iceberg may create a nice neat parcel but tastes of virtually nothing!

Many of my suggested 'fillings' include nuts and/or seeds but for those that don't or if you are creating your own combinations, I have also added a selection of nut and seed mixes that you can include or have on the side.

Suggestions (all tried and tested and tasty!)

Tinned salmon, chopped boiled egg, sliced mixed olives, sliced avocado, sliced cucumber, natural yoghurt, lemon juice and a good dash of smoked paprika powder.

Cold or hot sliced chicken, sautéed onions, garlic and ginger, sliced avocado, French dressing and toasted walnuts.

Parma ham, sautéed mushrooms, grilled or fresh tomato, scrambled egg or sliced boiled egg and Worcestershire sauce.

Cooked minced beef or lamb, fresh mint leaves, fresh coriander, sautéed onion and red chilli pepper and fish sauce (nam pla).

Firm tofu cubes sautéed until crisp in flavoured oil, sautéed onions, garlic, ginger and lemongrass, natural yoghurt, lime juice and toasted sesame seeds.

Sliced beef (hot or cold), tzatziki, toasted flaked almonds, lots of fresh mint and a drizzle of honey.

Hot or cold cooked prawns, sautéed garlic, red or yellow pepper, ginger and lemongrass, chopped fresh coriander, lime juice, natural yoghurt and toasted peanuts.

Hot or cold cooked chicken or turkey, sautéed spring onions and yellow peppers, grated hard cheese, freshly chopped parsley and toasted flaked almonds.

Minute steak or fillet steak, grilled and finely sliced, coarse grain mustard, sweet chilli sauce, sautéed mushrooms and spring onions, toasted cashew nuts.

Fresh prawns or crabmeat, cucumber, chopped boiled egg, yoghurt and toasted pine nuts.

Tinned tuna, coarse grain mustard, lime/lemon juice, anchovy sauce, sliced tomato and Greek yoghurt.

Many of the above suggestions include nuts and/or seeds but if not, here are a few nut and seed mixes that I recommend you add to your lunch - either scattered over your lettuce wraps or on the side.

NUT AND SEED MIXES

There is so much you can do with nuts and seeds and you will have noticed that they feature in a great many of my meals and snacks!

The quick and easy route is to buy large bags of mixed nuts and seeds, transfer them to small bags and store them in the fridge so you can grab one for snacking or topping or incorporating into recipes but I am not entirely convinced that all of them together make for a perfect marriage.

I prefer to buy them in separate packs and create my own mixes. These can then be portioned raw or toasted/roasted. I like to have 3 lidded jam jars at the back of the fridge which I keep topping up with my favourite mixes - saves time and money!

Roasted and toasted gets my vote but I also add in some fresh varieties straight from the pack.

If you are roasting nuts and seeds, pre-heat the oven to 180C/350F/ Gas Mark 4, place your selection in a high-sided roasting tray (this allows you to shake them around and spread them evenly without them ending up on the kitchen floor!) and bake in the middle of the oven for 5 minutes. Remove, give them a good shake and return for another 2 to 5 minutes or until they all have a nice crunch (use a timer as they go from 'nearly there' to burnt in the blink of an eye!)

If you are toasting nuts and seeds, preheat a non-stick frying pan over a medium heat, add your selection, shake the pan regularly, have a cold plate to hand and the second they start to brown around the edges, tip them out.

You can also crush your mixes very briefly in a spice grinder or mortar and pestle.

Here are 3 splendid combinations for your 3 jam jars to have 'at the ready' in the fridge:

roasted or toasted almonds, pine nuts, Brazil nuts and pumpkin seeds plus fresh pecans

roasted or toasted cashews, pistachios, walnuts and sunflower seeds plus fresh peanuts roasted or toasted peanuts, flaked almonds and coconut flakes with hemp hearts straight from the pack

You can also grind up all sorts of seeds (chia, sesame, hemp, flax etc) and add to your mixes.

SUSHI/SASHIMI + A CUP OR MUG OF SOUP

SUSHI/SASHIMI

It's confession time! I have tried to make my own sushi on a number of occasions but I don't seem to have the nimble fingers (or patience) required - they taste good but look like a bit of a road accident! Even when I came across Sonoko Sakai's delightful, idiot-proof, step-by-step article on the Lucky Peach blog it was still a step too far it seems! Have a look if you fancy having a go.

Sashimi however, is a different matter! I am in the enviable position of living just minutes away from a number of excellent fishmongers where I can get the very freshest, just-hours-off-the-boat Scottish produce (essential when it comes to sashimi) so when I have time to scoot down, I very quickly have one of the healthiest lunches imaginable - and - the accompanying sauces are quick and easy!

I serve the very, very finely sliced raw fish and shellfish (a frighteningly-sharp knife is a must here) alongside a salad of grated radish (or daikon if I can get it), grated carrot, grated courgette and grated tart apple and one or two of the following sauces or if time is really tight, a small bowl of dipping sauce from one of the local delis:

2 tablespoons tamari, ½ teaspoon dry mustard and 1 teaspoon sugar, mixed

1 tablespoon tamari, dash of rice wine vinegar, pinch of sugar, ¼ teaspoon finely grated fresh ginger, ¼ teaspoon peanut or sesame oil, 1 clove garlic, finely minced, pinch of cayenne pepper

1 teaspoon green wasabi mustard mixed with a little water and 1 tablespoon tamari

OFF THE SHELF SUSHI

Keep the following in mind:

- ideally the sushi will include some fresh ingredients. If it is simply smoked or cooked fish or just vegetables, this is a relatively good indication that it was not made that day.

- the shorter the shelf life, the better the sushi - plus - remember to remove your sushi from the fridge about half an hour before eating if you bought it in the morning. If it's too cold, the delicate tastes will be lost.

- you generally get what you pay for. The more expensive it is the greater likelihood the fish is fresh and not smoked.

OFF THE SHELF SASHIMI

Sashimi doesn't have a 'shelf life' so stick to outlets and restaurants where you know it comes in fresh every day.

A CUP OR MUG OF SOUP

Choose from the following and see recipes

- *Pea, Mint and Lettuce Soup*
- *Spinach and Watercress Soup*
- *Parsley Soup with Nuggets*
- *Silky-Smooth Celery Soup*
- *Blazing Hot Tomato Soup*
- *Spicy Turkey Soup*

Evening Meal Choices

Chicken and Barley Broth

(makes 4 bowls)

INGREDIENTS

- 1 small fresh chicken or 1 small ready-roasted chicken
- 20 cherry tomatoes
- 2 tablespoons light olive oil
- I medium onion, peeled and finely sliced
- 4 celery stalks, finely sliced
- 3 carrots, peeled and sliced or diced
- 1.5 litres chicken stock
- 5 small sprigs fresh thyme
- 150g barley, rinsed
- 150g green split peas, rinsed
- Sea salt and freshly ground black pepper
- 1 bag spinach leaves, roughly chopped

METHOD

Roast the chicken until cooked through, allow to cool slightly then remove the skin and chop the flesh into bite-sized pieces or remove the skin from the ready-roasted chicken and do the same.

Roast the tomatoes in a low oven for around 15 minutes or until they start to caramelise around the edges then remove from the oven and let them cool.

Warm the oil in a soup pot, add the onion, celery and carrot and gently sauté until just tender, about 8-10 minutes.

Add the stock and thyme, stir in the barley and split peas, bring to the boil then reduce the heat, cover and simmer for 25-30 minutes or until the barley and split peas are tender but still have a slight 'bite'.

Remove the thyme sprigs, check the seasoning then add the chicken flesh, the roasted tomatoes and the spinach.

Stir everything very gently making sure the tomatoes don't break up too much then simmer for a further 5-10 minutes.

Check the seasoning again and serve.

Like all broths, the longer you leave them, the thicker they become so add boiling water before serving to achieve desired consistency.

~

Barley packs a mighty punch nutritionally and has a lovely nutty taste - try this filling and brightly-coloured broth!

Roasted Red Pepper, Tomato and Chorizo Soup

(makes 4 bowls)

INGREDIENTS

- 1 red onion, skin on, quartered
- 2 long sweet red peppers, de-seeded and halved lengthways
- 4 fresh plum tomatoes, halved
- 2 garlic cloves, unpeeled
- 500ml chicken or vegetable stock
- Sea salt and freshly ground black pepper
- 400g can red kidney or cannellini beans, drained and rinsed
- 100g chorizo/smoked sausage, sliced
- 2 teaspoons Balsamic vinegar
- 15g fresh basil or parsley leaves, roughly chopped

METHOD

Preheat the grill to high. Arrange the onion, peppers and tomatoes on a baking sheet, cut sides down with the garlic cloves.

Grill the vegetables for 6-8 minutes or until the skins are beginning to blacken. Remove the skins from the onion, peppers and tomatoes and squeeze the garlic flesh from the skins (you can keep the skins on the peppers and tomatoes if time is tight!)

Chop half the vegetables into small chunks and put the remainder into a food processor or blender with the garlic flesh and stock. Blitz until smooth, then place in a soup pot with the chopped vegetables.

Season and heat the soup through until just boiling, stirring occasionally before reducing the heat, adding the beans, chorizo and Balsamic vinegar, covering and simmering gently for 5-7 minutes or until the chorizo is cooked through.

Toss in the basil/parsley and serve.

It also works well if you skin/peel and chop all the vegetables and sauté them in 1 tablespoon of light olive oil instead of roasting.

~

Tomato and red pepper always sit very comfortably together but when you roast them, marry them with beans, Balsamic vinegar, spicy chorizo and a handful of pungent herbs, the combination of flavours is pretty spectacular.

Lamb, Rice and Spinach Broth

(makes 4 bowls)

INGREDIENTS

- 1 tablespoon light olive oil
- 1 large onion, peeled and chopped/sliced
- 2 cloves garlic, peeled and crushed
- 1 teaspoon sea salt
- 500g lamb mince
- 750ml lamb or vegetable stock

- 1 x 400g tin chopped tomatoes
- 150g pre-cooked brown rice
- 1 tablespoon Worcestershire sauce
- Freshly ground black pepper
- 200g fresh spinach leaves

METHOD

Warm the oil in a soup pot, add the onion, garlic and salt, stir well, cover and sauté over a very low heat until the onion is pale and soft - around 15 minutes.

Meanwhile, in a hot pan, brown the minced lamb, stirring constantly until the pink colour disappears and it is slightly crisped around the edges. Remove from the heat, cover and set aside.

Add the stock and tomatoes to the soup pot, bring just to the boil, lower the heat and simmer for 5 minutes before adding the lamb (with its juices) and simmering for a further 5 minutes.

Add the rice, Worcestershire sauce and a few good grindings of black pepper and simmer for a further 10 minutes then add the spinach and continue simmering until it has just wilted but is still bright green.

If the soup is a little thick for your liking, add more stock or water.

Check the seasoning, adding more salt, pepper and/or Worcestershire sauce to taste.

If you make the soup ahead of time and either refrigerate or freeze it you will likely have to add more stock or water as the rice will swell and absorb quite a bit of the liquid.

NB: instead of lamb mince and lamb stock you can use beef mince and beef stock, chicken/turkey mince with chicken stock or use vegetable stock with whichever mince you choose.

~

This soup is a brilliant combination of protein, good fats, vegetables and just enough starchy carbohydrates to keep you firing on all cylinders for a few hours. I regard it as a superb meal-in-a bowl soup and many of my 'fitness enthusiastic' followers tell me it makes a superb post-exercise meal but that a small bowl just isn't enough!

Chicken, Chorizo and Greens Soup

(makes 4 bowls)

INGREDIENTS

- 1 large chicken portion (with leg and breast, skin on) or 2 chicken thighs and 2 chicken breasts, skin on - you can use ready-cooked chicken if time is tight
- 100g chorizo, finely sliced
- 1 tablespoon light olive oil
- 1 onion, peeled and finely chopped/sliced
- 2 cloves garlic, peeled and crushed
- 1 teaspoon sea salt
- 2 medium floury potatoes, peeled and diced
- 750ml chicken stock
- 1 head spring greens, cleaned, white cores removed and roughly chopped or two thirds of a bag of ready-chopped spring greens
- Sea salt and freshly ground black pepper
- Extra virgin olive oil
- Parmesan or Pecorino cheese (optional)

METHOD

Roast the chicken in the middle of a medium to hot oven until the skins are crisp and the flesh is cooked through then set aside, covered to cool slightly.

Very gently sauté the chorizo in a dry soup pot until the oils are released and the chorizo is crisp but not dried out. Remove the chorizo from the pot with a slotted spoon and set aside on kitchen paper.

Add the light olive oil to the oils that have been released from the chorizo and warm through before adding the onion, garlic and salt. Cover and leave to sauté over a very low heat for 20-30 minutes without browning until the onions are really soft.

Add the potatoes and half the stock, bring to the boil, turn the heat to low, cover and simmer for about 10-15 minutes or until the potatoes are cooked through.

Add the greens and the rest of the stock to the pot and continue simmering for 5-10 minutes or until the greens are just cooked through.

Meanwhile, remove the skin from the chicken and dice, slice or shred the flesh before adding to the pot along with the chorizo. The liquid should just cover the ingredients so you may need to add a little boiling water.

Keep simmering over a low heat until everything is piping hot, check the seasoning and gently mash the soup with a potato masher until some of the potato and chorizo are slightly mushy - or to your desired consistency. Add more stock or water if necessary.

Serve with a good drizzle of extra virgin olive oil and a generous grating of Parmesan or Pecorino cheese.

~

Only thing I can say about this soup is that you really have to make it - it's top dollar and very moreish!

Curry Soup

(makes 4 bowls)

INGREDIENTS

- 100g white basmati rice
- 100ml chicken or vegetable stock
- 200ml full cream milk
- 2 tablespoons coconut oil
- 1 teaspoon mustard seeds
- ½ teaspoon fenugreek seeds
- ½ teaspoon cumin seeds
- 3 dried red chillies, crushed
- 6 shallots, peeled and finely chopped

- 1 teaspoon peeled and grated fresh ginger
- 5 cloves garlic, peeled and crushed
- 2 green chillies, de-seeded and finely chopped
- 10 curry leaves
- ½ teaspoon turmeric powder
- Sea salt
- 1 red chilli, de-seeded and finely diced
- Fresh coriander leaves, finely chopped

METHOD

Place the stock and 120ml of the milk in a medium-sized pot, bring just to the boil, turn the heat to the lowest possible setting, add the rice, stir well, cover the pot with a tight-fitting lid and cook for 10 minutes then turn the heat off completely and let the rice sit while you make the soup - don't remove the lid!

Meanwhile, warm the oil in a soup pot over a medium heat and toss in the seeds and dry red chillies. Stir well and let them 'pop' and infuse for a minute or two.

Add the shallots, ginger, garlic, green chillies and curry leaves and sauté everything gently until the shallots are soft but not browned.

Add the turmeric followed by the rice then while continuing to stir over a low heat, add the rest of the milk and keep stirring until it just begins to bubble (don't let it boil) then turn the heat off.

Check the seasoning, remove the curry leaves and serve topped with the red chilli sautéed in a little oil plus the coriander leaves.

NB: As rice soaks up liquid like a sponge, you may need to add some boiling water or a little more stock to get the consistency that suits you.

~

This soup is a glorious colour, is very filling, is rich in metabolism-boosting spices and packs a real punch!

Creamy Tomato and Bacon Soup

(makes 4 bowls)

INGREDIENTS

- 1 tablespoon light olive oil
- 1 medium onion, peeled and finely chopped
- 8 rashers smoked lean bacon, chopped into bite-sized chunks
- 1 dessertspoon cornflour
- 1 x 400g tin chopped tomatoes
- 1 teaspoon sugar
- Sea salt and freshly ground black pepper
- 250ml good quality chicken stock
- 250ml full-cream milk

METHOD

Warm the oil in a soup pot and gently sauté the onion until translucent and very, very soft.

Increase the heat slightly, add the bacon and continue to sauté for a few minutes, stirring all the time until the edges of both the onion and the bacon are slightly caramelised.

Reduce the heat again, stir in the cornflour and cook for another 5 minutes then add the tinned tomatoes, sugar (hey it's only one teaspoon between 4 bowls!), a good pinch of sea salt and at least 5 good twists of black pepper and continue to cook on a low heat for 5-6 minutes.

Add the stock, stir well, increase the heat, bring the soup to just boiling then reduce the heat to a very low setting.

After about 5 minutes, add the milk and keep stirring until the soup is hot and ready to serve (don't let it boil or the milk will curdle).

~

I have been making this soup since I was a 'teen learning to cook', it has always been a staple in my household, kids love it (particularly when you blitz it in a blender). It's quick, filling and delicious, what more can I say?

One-Pot Chicken, Fish or Chickpeas

(makes 2 servings)

INGREDIENTS

- 200g peeled and diced sweet potato
- 3 cloves garlic, unpeeled
- 2 organic chicken thighs, skin on or 2 fish fillets or 200g tinned chickpeas, drained and rinsed
- 40ml chicken or vegetable stock
- ¼ lemon cut into 2 wedges
- 1 tablespoon light avocado or olive oil
- Sea salt and freshly ground black pepper
- 1 small courgette, wiped and cut into good-sized chunks
- ½ red chilli, de-seeded and finely sliced
- 50g chorizo, sliced
- ½ small bag baby spinach leaves
- 1 tablespoon chopped fresh parsley leaves

METHOD

Preheat the oven to 220C/425F/Gas Mark 7

Spread the sweet potato and garlic over the base of a small, deep roasting tin and place the chicken (skin side up) on top.

Pour the stock in, pop the lemon wedges around the tin, drizzle the oil over the whole lot, season with a good pinch of salt and lots of pepper and place the roasting tin (uncovered) in the middle of the oven for 20 minutes.

Remove the tin from the oven and add the courgette, chilli and chorizo, mix everything well but still keep the chicken (skin side up) on top and return to the oven for another 20 to 30 minutes or until the chicken is cooked through and the vegetables are 'al dente'.

Remove the tin from the oven again, squeeze the flesh from the garlic cloves, mix it through and discard the skins before stuffing the spinach and parsley leaves in and around everything - seems like there is way too much but they soon wilt - then return to the oven for 5 to 10 minutes before serving.

NB: If using fish or chickpeas instead of chicken, wait until 15 to 20 minutes before the end of the cooking time before adding them. You can also omit the chorizo if you are not a meat-eater.

~

I love a one-pot dish that does it's own thing in the oven! Preparation time is quick and you can get on with a pile of tasks whilst the cooking happens...

Quinoa Vegetable Bake

(makes 4 servings)

INGREDIENTS

- 1 tablespoon coconut oil
- 1 small onion, peeled and finely chopped/sliced
- 1 small courgette/zucchini, wiped and diced
- 1 small carrot, peeled and diced/roughly grated
- 1 small red pepper, de-seeded and finely chopped
- 6 sun dried tomatoes in oil, drained and roughly chopped
- 1 garlic clove, peeled and crushed
- 1 teaspoon sea salt
- Freshly ground black pepper
- 125g baby spinach leaves
- 1 heaped tablespoon chopped parsley leaves
- 100g quinoa, thoroughly rinsed
- 2 heaped tablespoons natural cottage cheese
- 1 egg, lightly beaten

METHOD

Preheat the oven to 180C/350F/Gas Mark 4.

Warm the coconut oil in a deep sauté pan, add the onion, courgette, carrot, red pepper, tomatoes, garlic, salt and pepper and mix well.

Cover the pan and sauté over a very gentle heat until all the vegetables are cooked through but still have a bit of bite (15 to 20 minutes).

Stir in the spinach and continue to cook until the leaves have just wilted then turn off the heat.

Stir in the parsley, quinoa, cottage cheese and egg and thoroughly mix before transferring to a shallow ovenproof dish.

Bake, uncovered until the egg is just set - around 45 minutes but check after 35 minutes by using a skewer - it will come out clean when the egg is set. Serve with a green salad.

~

A brilliant 'bake' that has everything going for it! Keeps well in the fridge for a day and can be reheated .....and is seriously filling and tasty!

Mediterranean Vegetable Bake

(makes 4 servings)

INGREDIENTS

- 1½ tablespoons avocado oil
- 1 medium onion, peeled and finely chopped
- 2 cloves garlic, peeled and crushed
- 1 medium red pepper, de-seeded and diced
- 1 medium yellow pepper, de-seeded and diced
- 1 small red chilli, de-seeded and very finely diced
- 2 medium courgette/zucchini, washed and diced
- 3 tablespoons finely chopped parsley leaves
- 1 tablespoon fresh basil leaves, finely chopped

- 1 teaspoon dried oregano or marjoram
- 200g cooked brown rice
- 150g ricotta cheese
- 150g feta cheese, crumbled
- 1 tablespoon fresh lemon juice
- Sea salt and freshly ground black pepper
- 6 medium tomatoes, sliced
- 10 black olives, stoned and halved

METHOD

Preheat the oven to 190C/375F/Gas Mark 5 and place a non-stick baking dish on the middle shelf.

Heat the oil in a sauté pan over a medium heat, add the onion, garlic, peppers and chilli, stir well, turn the heat to very low, put a lid on the pan and sauté for around 10 minutes or until the vegetables are cooked through.

Remove the pan from the heat, stir in the courgette/zucchini and herbs and set aside.

Place the rice, ricotta, feta and lemon juice in a bowl and mix well. Add the vegetables from the pan and continue mixing gently until everything is incorporated.

Season to taste and turn the mixture into the heated baking dish, smoothing the surface flat before topping with the tomato slices (slightly overlap them), sprinkling the olive halves over evenly and returning to the oven for 35-45 minutes or until everything is piping hot.

If you wish, you can then place the dish under the grill for a further 5 minutes to slightly crisp the edges of the tomatoes.

~

This dish is a real feast of vegetables but also rich in protein, good fats and starch making it a beautifully-balanced and satisfying meal... it is also great cold alongside a generous mixed, dressed green salad.

Parcel-Baked Fish

(makes 1 serving)

INGREDIENTS

- 1 white fish fillet
- 1 generous handful fresh spinach leaves
- 1 small onion, peeled and very finely sliced into rings
- 6 fresh asparagus tips
- 1 tomato, sliced
- 1 small red chilli, de-seeded and finely sliced (optional)
- 1 tablespoon chopped fresh parsley or coriander
- 2 teaspoons lemon juice
- 2 teaspoons avocado or light olive oil
- Sea salt and freshly ground black pepper

METHOD

Preheat the oven to 200C/400F/Gas Mark 6.

Lay out one piece of aluminium foil about 12-14 inches square and place the spinach on it.

Lay the fish fillet on the bed of spinach followed by the onion, asparagus, tomato, chilli (if using) and herbs. Drizzle the lemon juice and oil over and season lightly with salt and pepper.

Fold the foil to create a parcel, leaving plenty of space around the contents, place on a baking sheet and bake for around 25 minutes or until the fish is cooked and the juices run clear.

Timing will depend on the thickness of the fish fillet so take a peek after 25 minutes. Be careful when opening the foil as hot steam will escape.

When cooked, lift the contents of the parcel onto a warmed plate and spoon over the delicious juices.

~

Fish was born to be baked in a parcel. All the juices meld together creating a delicious, quick and super-healthy meal. Buy fish and vegetables in season and add herbs and spices to sharpen things up.

Crispy-Topped Baked Fish

(makes 1 serving)

INGREDIENTS

- 1 white fish fillet or
- 1 slice tofu (around 2cm thick) or 1 medium-sized skinless chicken breast
- 1 tablespoon oats
- 1 tablespoon fresh parsley, finely chopped
- 1 tablespoon lemon juice
- Sea salt and freshly ground black pepper
- 2 teaspoons light olive or coconut oil
- 3 spring onions, trimmed and finely sliced
- 2 heaped teaspoons tomato purée
- 1 medium-sized tomato, sliced
- 15g Parmesan cheese, grated

METHOD

Preheat the oven to 200C/400F/Gas Mark 6.

In a small bowl, mix the oats, parsley and lemon juice, lightly season and set aside.

Warm the oil in a small sauté pan and cook the spring onions over a medium heat until soft then add the tomato purée and mix well.

For fish or tofu: Place a sheet of baking foil in a small oven-proof dish, place the fish or tofu in the middle and pull up the sides of the foil so you create an open-topped parcel.

Top the fish/tofu with the spring onion/tomato purée mix, arrange the tomato slices on top and finally the oat mix (don't close the parcel) then place the dish on a middle shelf in the oven and bake until cooked through.

Thin fish fillets and tofu will take around 5-6 minutes, thicker/denser fish fillets will take around 8-12 minutes. Have a peek and check that the fish flakes nicely and the juice runs clear.

Remove from the oven, turn the oven off and the grill on (to a medium heat), scatter the cheese on top, grill on the lowest shelf until the cheese melts and is just beginning to brown (around 5 minutes) then with a fish slice, lift the fish/tofu onto a warmed serving plate and spoon over the cooking juices.

For the chicken: Place the chicken on the foil, lightly season, add a splash of oil, scrunch the foil so it creates a loose but sealed parcel and bake for 10 minutes then open up the parcel, top as per the fish/tofu and bake for a further 10 minutes or until the juices run clear and the chicken is cooked through. Continue as before and serve.

~

The tasty topping can be made in advance, making this dish a real 'no brainer' when you're tight for time.

MEAL IN A BOWL SALADS

Smoked Bacon and Queenie Salad

(makes 1 serving)

INGREDIENTS

- 2 thick rashers smoked streaky bacon
- 1 tablespoon light olive oil
- Splash of red wine/sherry vinegar
- Splash of Balsamic vinegar
- 4 queen scallops
- 4 thin asparagus spears
- 1 free range, organic egg for poaching
- Parmesan cheese for grating
- Sea salt and freshly ground black pepper
- Mixed salad leaves

METHOD

Fry the bacon rashers over a medium heat in their own fat until crisp. Remove and reserve but keep just a trace of the fat in the pan for cooking the scallops.

In a small pan, place the oil, the red wine/sherry vinegar, the Balsamic, a scant pinch of salt and a few grindings of black pepper. Heat through, but do not allow to boil.

Meanwhile, lightly steam the asparagus spears and poach the egg.

Season the scallops very lightly with salt, add to the pan with the scant covering of bacon fat and fry quickly for 45 seconds to 1 minute on each side depending on their size. Do not overcook or they will become rubbery.

Stir the scallops and bacon into the warm dressing, arrange a small pile of salad leaves in the centre of a plate or bowl and spoon the scallops and bacon over the top. Place the poached egg on top and scatter the asparagus spears around.

Drizzle any remaining dressing over the salad, generously grate over some fresh Parmesan and serve immediately.

~

At last! The salad that features on the cover of the book! If you are a shellfish lover, this is way, way, way better than even delicious, it's one of those salads you just have to keep repeating and repeating. It also works well with lightly sautéed chicken or duck 'bites' or crispy oven-baked tofu cubes and if you struggle with poaching eggs, a soft boiled egg is a good alternative.

Greek Salad with a Difference!

(makes 2 servings)

INGREDIENTS

SPICY FETA CHEESE:

- 100g feta, cut into bite sized chunks
- ½ teaspoon cumin seeds
- ½ teaspoon fennel seeds
- 1 tablespoon cold-pressed extra virgin olive oil, preferably Greek

SALAD:

- ½ sweet potato, cut into 1 inch cubes
- Light olive oil for roasting
- ¼ aubergine, cut into 1 inch cubes
- 50g black olives, stoned and halved
- ½ medium red onion, peeled and very thinly sliced
- 3 tomatoes, cut into large chunks
- ¼ cucumber, cut into bite sized chunks
- 1 level teaspoon dried oregano
- 2 tablespoons fresh lemon juice
- 1 tablespoon cold-pressed extra virgin olive oil
- Sea salt and freshly ground black pepper

METHOD

Preheat the oven to 200C/400F/Gas Mark 6.

Toast the fennel and cumin seeds for a minute or so in a dry pan until the aromas are released.

Combine the seeds with the feta and extra virgin olive oil in a bowl, making sure the feta is coated in the spiced oil. Place in the fridge for as long as possible to marinate (overnight is great).

Place the sweet potatoes on a baking tray and drizzle with a little of the light olive oil. Roast in the oven for 35 minutes then add the aubergine and roast for a further 10 to 15 minutes then allow them to cool a little while you prepare the salad.

Combine the olives, red onion, tomatoes, cucumber, oregano, lemon juice and extra virgin olive oil in a bowl, mix in the marinated feta, add the sweet potato and aubergine and toss everything together before serving.

~

The 'spicing' of the feta and the addition of the sweet potatoes and aubergine make this a really fresh but very filling salad. It can also be made earlier in the day and kept, covered in the fridge - just remember to take it out and allow it to come to room temperature before eating to maximise the flavours.

Spiced Lamb Salad

(makes 2 servings)

INGREDIENTS

FOR THE NUT, SEED AND SPICE MIX:
- 50g fresh hazelnuts
- 40g sesame seeds
- 1 tablespoon coriander seeds
- 1 tablespoon cumin seeds
- ½ teaspoon coarsely ground black pepper
- ½ teaspoon sea salt crystals

FOR THE SALAD:
- Zest and juice of ½ lemon
- 1 tablespoon Manuka honey
- 30ml extra virgin olive oil
- Sea salt and freshly ground black pepper
- 60g couscous
- 75ml boiling water
- ½ tablespoon light olive oil or coconut oil

- 250g lean lamb fillet in one piece
- Large slice watermelon, skinned, de-seeded and sliced or diced
- 75g Greek feta cheese, crudely crumbled
- Generous handful fresh watercress leaves

METHOD

Dry fry the hazelnuts in a shallow sauté pan over a medium heat until they are golden brown and crunchy (watch them, they have a nasty habit of burning when you take your eye off them!)

Immediately put them between a few sheets of kitchen roll and rub vigorously until most of the outer skins come off then transfer them to a mortar and pestle or spice grinder and bash/grind until they are coarsely chopped.

In the same pan, toast the sesame seeds until golden before adding to the hazelnuts.

In the same pan, toast the coriander and cumin seeds until they start to 'pop' before transferring them to a mortar and pestle or grinder and blitzing until they are finely crushed then add them to the hazelnut/sesame seed mix.

Add the salt and pepper, mix and set aside. Whisk the lemon zest, lemon juice, honey and extra virgin olive oil in a bowl, season to taste and set aside.

Put the couscous in a medium-sized bowl, gradually pour over the boiling water, mixing with a fork all the time, cover and leave for around 10 minutes.

Heat the light olive oil or coconut oil in a sauté pan and over a relatively high heat, brown the lamb fillet on all sides before turning down the heat and continuing to cook for a further 5 minutes if you like it pink, 8 minutes if you like it medium and 10 minutes if you like it well-done. Turn the fillet occasionally.

Remove the lamb from the pan, spread the nut, seed and spice mix on a board and roll the lamb in it until it is well-coated before wrapping in foil to keep warm.

Fork through the couscous to separate all grains before adding the lemon/honey/oil mix and stirring to ensure it is well incorporated.

Place a portion of couscous on each plate, top with the lamb (very thinly sliced) and arrange the feta, watermelon and watercress around the plate.

The nut, seed and spice mix will keep in the fridge in a sealed jar for a week if you choose to make it beforehand or double the quantities and makes a delicious soup, stew, salad and bruschetta or crisp bread topping.

~

The combination of lean, slightly pink lamb, watermelon and feta cheese is already a winner but add the nut, seed and spice mix and this becomes way more than just any old salad - it quickly becomes a household staple (and is equally good cold as it stays fresh and delicious for hours in a sealed container)!

Warm Salad with Haggis

(makes 2 servings

INGREDIENTS

- 3 heaped teaspoons coarse grain mustard
- 6 tablespoons extra virgin cold-pressed olive oil
- 1 tablespoon white wine vinegar
- Sea salt
- Freshly ground black pepper
- 1 x 130g packet 'microwave in 60 seconds' traditional or vegetarian haggis or 130g black pudding or a mix of both
- 100g baby salad leaves
- ½ Granny Smith apple, peeled, cored and finely diced
- 50g red onion, peeled and very finely sliced

METHOD

To make the dressing, whisk the mustard and vinegar together, blend in the oil, season and put to one side.

Heat the haggis in the microwave or grill the black pudding (or both), arrange the salad leaves on the plates, gently pour over the dressing, break up the haggis/black pudding, place on top of the leaves and garnish with the apple and red onion.

~

Okay, I get why non meat eaters, vegetarians and vegans don't 'do' haggis but as for the rest - you don't know what you are missing - this is one supremely tasty and satisfying little addition to meat-eaters diets!

*I include this recipe with the kind permission of Jo Macsween, the driving force behind Macsween of Edinburgh **www.macsween. co.uk** who, in my view make simply the best haggis in the world. She published The Macsween Haggis Bible, a delightful little book which addresses haggis mysteries, quashes a few haggis myths and offers an inspiring selection of recipes which show haggis off at its very best... this salad is one that ticks a whole load of fat busting boxes and is knock-out!*

VERY QUICK DINNERS

Very Quick Salmon

(makes 1 serving)

Lightly paint a salmon fillet or salmon steak with olive oil and grill under a moderate heat for 7-8 minutes, turning once. Sprinkle with Worcestershire Sauce or Balsamic vinegar and lime or lemon juice just before serving with at least 3 steamed or roasted vegetables or a lightly-dressed mixed salad.

Very Quick Lamb

(makes 1 serving)

Rub a lamb steak with lemon zest, a pinch of cinnamon and a splash of olive oil mixed. Grill under a moderate heat for 4 minutes each side if you like it pink, longer for well done. Put on a warm plate and leave to rest for a few minutes while you heat through a little fresh orange juice with very finely diced red chilli then pour this over the lamb. Serve with at least 3 steamed or roasted vegetables or a lightly-dressed mixed salad.

Very Quick Chicken

(makes 1 serving)

Steam a skinless chicken breast either on a plate (cover it loosely with tinfoil/greaseproof paper) over a pot of simmering water or in a steam basket for 10-15 minutes until cooked through. Spread pesto or olive paste on top and put under the grill (low heat) for a couple of minutes until bubbling. Serve with at least 3 steamed or roasted vegetables or a lightly-dressed mixed salad.

Very Quick Burger

(makes 1 serving)

Use freshly ground lean beef or soya mince which has been soaked as per packet instructions. Add some sea salt crystals, ground black pepper and other spices of choice, plus a few shakes of Worcestershire Sauce or Balsamic vinegar. Mould into burger shapes and chill for 15 minutes before grilling. Top with a slice of goats cheese or cheddar towards the end of cooking until melted and bubbling (optional). Serve with at least 3 steamed or roasted vegetables or a lightly-dressed mixed salad.

Very Quick Prawns

(makes 1 serving)

Coat half a dozen large, fresh, shelled prawns with chilli, garlic or lemon-infused olive oil and grill both sides until pink but not dried out (2-6 minutes depending on the size of the prawns). Serve with at least 3 steamed or roasted vegetables or a lightly-dressed mixed salad.

Very Quick Tofu

(makes 1 serving)

Cut firm tofu into cubes and stir fry quickly in a little olive oil mixed with crushed garlic and grated fresh ginger. Add a squeeze of runny honey and top with toasted flaked almonds. Serve with at least 3 steamed or roasted vegetables or a lightly-dressed mixed salad.

Singapore-Style Noodles

(makes 1 serving)

INGREDIENTS

- Frozen mixed vegetables
- Frozen peas and corn
- Egg noodles
- 5 spice powder and mild curry powder
- Soy sauce or mirin
- Sweet chilli sauce
- Beansprouts

METHOD

Cook a good handful of egg noodles according to the packet instructions.

Cook at least 4 handfuls of frozen vegetables according to packet instructions.

Put the whole lot in a wide shallow pan, add a good pinch of 5 spice powder, a good pinch of curry powder, a good splash of soy sauce or mirin and a small teaspoon of sweet chilli sauce and stir everything vigorously until nicely mixed then add a handful of beansprouts just at the end and give it another good stir before serving.

~

This is a dish for those days when you hit the kitchen at dinner time and it has to be all about what is in the fridge, freezer and cupboard but that doesn't mean the diet has to go awry or you can't get a whole load of nourishment into your exhausted frame - just make sure you always have the above ingredients in stock and it's all good... it's all quick... it's all easy and... it's super tasty!

CURRIES AND CASSEROLES

Aubergine Curry with Meat, Poultry, Fish or Legumes

(makes 4 servings)

INGREDIENTS

- 1 ripe mango, peeled, stoned and diced
- 1 teaspoon sugar
- 2 tablespoons finely chopped mint leaves
- Sea salt
- Fresh lemon juice
- 1 tablespoon light olive oil
- 450g fresh, skinless chicken breasts cut into bite-sized pieces
- 1 tablespoon coconut oil
- 1 large or 2 small aubergines, wiped and cut into bite-sized chunks
- 225g button mushrooms, cleaned and halved
- 6-8 cherry tomatoes, halved
- 2 teaspoons peeled and grated fresh ginger
- 2 cloves garlic, peeled and grated/mashed
- 2 teaspoons curry powder
- 2 level tablespoons Thai red curry paste
- ½ teaspoon chilli flakes
- 2 heaped tablespoons 'no added sugar' almond butter
- 250ml unsweetened almond milk

- ½ x 400ml can coconut milk
- 240g tinned or jarred chickpeas, drained and rinsed
- 2 good handfuls roughly chopped coriander leaves
- 2 good handfuls roughly chopped basil leaves
- Raw cauliflower (white only) box-grated and steamed or microwaved for a couple of minutes

METHOD

The salsa: mix the mango, sugar, mint, a good pinch of salt and a couple of tablespoons of lemon juice together in a bowl, cover and set aside.

The curry: warm the olive oil in a large, shallow pan and sauté the chicken pieces until lightly-browned and just cooked through before removing them (and their juices) to a dish and setting aside.

Add the coconut oil to the pan, warm through then sauté the aubergine, mushrooms, tomatoes, ginger and garlic over a medium heat for 5 to 10 minutes.

Return the chicken pieces and their juices to the pan and continue to sauté for another few minutes, stirring carefully so as not to break up the vegetables.

Mix the curry powder, Thai curry paste, chilli flakes and almond butter into a cupful of the almond milk and stir well until very smooth then add this mix to the pan followed by the rest of the almond milk, the coconut milk and the chickpeas. Stir well, bring slowly to the boil then turn the heat to low and simmer for 5 minutes.

Just before serving, add the basil and coriander to the curry and stir to combine for a scant minute or two before serving on a bed of the cauliflower with the fresh mango salsa alongside (good quality mango chutney also works well).

NB: replace the chicken with the same amount of turkey, lean lamb, veal, firm white fish, fresh prawns or tofu (all cut into bite-sized chunks before sautéing in the olive oil until just cooked through as per the chicken).

ALSO: you can play around with the spices if you like your curry hotter or milder and add more or less of the almond butter.

~

This is truly amazingly good - one of my resident 'tasters' declared it the best curry she has ever had... and it tastes great with all the different protein choices making it a meal that can be regularly repeated without diet boredom creeping in! It also freezes well.

Aromatic Lamb/Beef Casserole

(makes 2 servings)

INGREDIENTS

- 2 tablespoons sesame seeds
- 400g lean lamb or beef, trimmed and cut into bite-sized pieces
- Lamb/beef stock
- 1 small onion, peeled and finely chopped
- 1 level tablespoon coconut oil
- ¼ teaspoon saffron powder
- ¼ teaspoon ground ginger
- ½ teaspoon ground coriander
- ½ teaspoon ground cinnamon
- Sea salt and freshly ground black pepper
- 1 tablespoon Manuka honey (optional)

METHOD

Toast the sesame seeds in a dry frying pan, tossing until golden then set aside (watch them as they burn very quickly).

Put the meat in a medium-sized pan, barely cover with stock and add the onion, oil, saffron, ginger, coriander and cinnamon.

Stir well, bring to the boil, cover the pan and simmer very gently until the meat is extremely tender and the liquid is a rich sauce (about 2 hours but check after an hour and a half and add more stock if required).

Season to taste, stir in the honey (if using) and simmer for a further 5 minutes. Cool and refrigerate/freeze at this stage if desired.

Garnish with toasted sesame seeds before serving with at least 3 steamed, stir fried or roasted vegetables or a lightly-dressed, mixed salad.

~

It's all about long, slow cooking here but as everything goes into the pot at once, it takes very little time to prepare and... it's even better if you leave it in the fridge for a day or freeze and bring it back to the table. Careful though, the temptation to mop up the juices with crusty bread can be hard to control!

Lemon Ginger Chicken

(makes 1 serving)

INGREDIENTS

- 3 skinless mini chicken fillets
- 1 tablespoon light olive or coconut oil
- ½ red onion, finely sliced
- 1 celery stick, peeled and finely sliced
- 2 large tomatoes, skinned, de-seeded and chopped or a small can (200ml) chopped tomatoes, sieved to remove the liquid
- 1 teaspoon peeled and grated fresh ginger
- 1 teaspoon lemon grass paste
- 1 tablespoon Balsamic vinegar
- 1 heaped tablespoon fresh coriander leaves, roughly chopped
- Sea salt and freshly ground black pepper
- ½ ripe avocado, stoned, peeled and roughly chopped
- 2 teaspoons lime or lemon juice
- Chilli powder (hot or mild)

METHOD

Preheat the oven to 200C/400F/Gas Mark 6.

Place the chicken fillets on a piece of baking foil large enough to form a loose parcel, lightly season, add a good splash of oil, scrunch all the edges of the foil together, place in an oven-proof baking dish and bake for 8-10 minutes or until the chicken is cooked through and the juices run clear then set aside, covered.

Warm the rest of the oil in a small sauté pan, add the onion and celery and cook gently until they are soft but not browned.

Add the tomato, ginger, lemon grass and vinegar, stir well and continue to cook over a medium heat until the vinegar starts to evaporate and the sauce becomes a thickish paste (around 5-7 minutes).

Add the coriander, season to taste, mix well, turn off the heat and place a lid on the pan.

In a small bowl, roughly mash the avocado with a fork, add the lime/lemon juice, lightly season and mix thoroughly.

To serve, spoon the sauce onto a warmed plate, place the chicken fillets, finely sliced on top and finally the avocado.

Lightly dust with chilli powder.

~

This was an experiment that really worked! The cool, creamy avocado topping married with the heat of the ginger and lemon grass and the sharpness of the lemon and vinegar takes the succulent chicken fillets to a whole new place.

Sweet Potato Curry

(makes 2 servings)

INGREDIENTS

- ½ tablespoon coconut oil
- ½ medium onion, peeled and finely sliced
- ½ clove garlic, peeled and crushed
- ½ teaspoon sea salt
- 1 level teaspoon curry powder
- ¼ teaspoon cayenne pepper
- ½ x 400g can pineapple pieces in fruit juice, drained and lightly crushed
- 1 medium sweet potato, peeled and cut into bite-sized chunks
- ½ x 400ml can coconut milk
- 2 very generous handfuls baby spinach leaves

METHOD

Heat the coconut oil in a deep sauté pan, add the onion, garlic and salt, stir briskly over a medium heat for a minute or two then turn the heat down to very low, place a lid on the pan and sauté for around 10 minutes or until the onion is soft.

Add the curry powder and cayenne pepper, stir well and sauté for a further 5 minutes before adding the sweet potato, stirring again, turning the heat up to medium and sautéing the whole mixture for a further 5 minutes.

Add the coconut milk and the pineapples, continue cooking until the mixture is lightly bubbling then turn the heat to very low, put the lid on and cook for a further 20-25 minutes or until the sweet potato is cooked through.

Add the spinach and stir well into the mix until just wilted and serve immediately.

~

Very quick, very tasty and just as hot or mild as you like your curries. Don't stint on the spinach - it seems like a lot when you add it but it wilts down fast and is bursting with essential vitamins and minerals - a veritable 'super' dish!

Venison Chilli

(makes 4 servings)

INGREDIENTS

- 1 tablespoon light olive oil or coconut oil
- ½ medium onion, peeled and finely chopped
- 1 clove garlic, peeled and crushed/minced
- 2 jalapeño peppers, de-seeded and diced
- 500g prime wild venison mince
- 2 tablespoons chilli powder
- 1 teaspoon ground cumin
- 1 teaspoon dried oregano
- 1 x 400g tin red kidney beans, drained and rinsed

- 1 x 400g tin black beans, drained and rinsed
- 60g corn, fresh or frozen
- 1 x 400g tin chopped tomatoes
- 4 tablespoons tomato purée
- Sea salt and freshly ground black pepper
- 2 tablespoons full fat crème fraîche
- 1 small fresh cauliflower, green leaves removed and florets roughly grated on a box grater
- Lots of coriander leaves, finely chopped
- 1 small red chilli, de-seeded and finely diced

METHOD

Warm the oil over a medium heat in a large thick-bottomed pot, add the onion and a teaspoon of sea salt crystals, turn the heat to very, very low, put a lid on the pot and very gently sauté until the onion is soft.

Add the garlic and peppers, stir well, cover and sauté for a further 5 minutes or until the peppers are beginning to soften.

In a separate pot, brown the venison mince over a high heat, stirring vigorously until every morsel of mince is nicely browned then add it to the onion/garlic/pepper mix, add the spices and stir well to combine.

Stir in the kidney beans, black beans, corn, tomatoes and tomato purée, bring just to the boil then reduce to a very gentle simmer, cover and cook for around an hour.

Before serving, remove the lid, turn up the heat and let the chilli bubble and reduce for around 15-20 minutes. Leave to cool a little then gently stir in the crème fraîche

Serve on a bed of raw cauliflower 'rice' mixed with coriander and diced red chilli (you can steam or microwave the cauliflower for a couple of minutes if you wish).

~

Great combo, no starch thanks to the cauliflower 'rice' and venison makes a brilliant, leaner alternative to beef and you can substitute natural yoghurt for the crème fraîche...

Poached Egg Special

(makes 1 serving)

INGREDIENTS

- ½ tablespoon coconut or olive oil
- 1 large 'beef' mushroom, stem removed and top peeled
- 1 large free range or *'happy'* egg
- A handful of fresh baby spinach leaves
- ½ avocado, stone out, peeled and sliced
- 2 thin slices smoked salmon or smoked ham
- Sea salt and freshly ground black pepper

METHOD

Warm the oil in a shallow pan over a medium heat then sauté the mushroom for around 5 minutes, turning regularly until well-browned and cooked through.

Remove from the heat, turn the mushroom, gill side up, lightly season, place the spinach leaves on top and cover with a lid or foil to keep warm (this allows the spinach to wilt a little).

Crack the egg into a teacup, bring a small pan of water to the boil, turn it down to barely bubbling, give it a good swirl with a whisk then slide the egg into the middle of the vortex and cook for 3 minutes before removing with a slotted spoon and placing it on a few sheets of kitchen towel to absorb excess water.

Place the mushroom/spinach on a warmed serving plate followed by the sliced avocado, smoked salmon or ham and finally the egg, season to taste and eat immediately.

~

This also works well with scrambled egg, a halved soft boiled egg or an egg fried in top quality butter if you find poaching eggs a bit stressful! This is a really great 'don't have time to think, just need to eat' dish!

Tofu Towers

(makes 1 serving)

INGREDIENTS

- 1 tablespoon sesame seeds
- 2 slices firm tofu (2-3cm thick)
- 1 tablespoon sweet chilli sauce
- ½ level teaspoon ground ginger
- ½ teaspoon coconut oil
- ½ teaspoon soy sauce
- 2 thick slices aubergine
- Light olive oil
- Sea salt and freshly ground black pepper
- 2 large eggs
- 2 large handfuls fresh spinach leaves

METHOD

Toss the sesame seeds in a pan over a medium heat until toasted and set aside.

Wrap the tofu slices in kitchen paper and press firmly to absorb most of the water.

Mix the chilli sauce, ginger, coconut oil and soy sauce and paint both sides of the tofu slices then put them under a hot grill or on a griddle pan and cook, turning regularly until they are golden.

Coat both sides of the aubergine slices with oil and season with salt and pepper before grilling or griddling as per the tofu. Turn regularly until cooked through and nut brown on both sides.

Keep the aubergine and tofu warm while you poach the eggs.

Quickly rinse the spinach leaves, microwave or steam until just wilting then dry the leaves in plenty of kitchen paper.

To serve, put the aubergine slices on a warmed plate followed by the tofu, the spinach, the poached eggs and finally the sesame seeds.

~

I can't remember where the inspiration for this recipe came from but aubergine, tofu and spices are a great combination and the runny egg completes the dish beautifully. I generally go for 2 eggs but you may prefer to just have one - depends on how hungry you are!

Mexican-Style Baked Omelette

(makes 3 servings)

INGREDIENTS

- 5cm piece chorizo, finely sliced
- A knob of top quality butter
- 1 small onion, peeled and finely sliced
- ½ long thin red pepper, de-seeded and finely sliced
- 6 brown-capped mushrooms, stalks removed, cleaned and finely sliced
- 2 medium-sized, ripe tomatoes
- 6 medium organic, free-range eggs
- 2 tablespoons grated goats cheddar or hard ewes milk cheese
- Sea salt and freshly ground black pepper

METHOD

Preheat the oven to 200C/400F/Gas Mark 6.

Skin your tomatoes by putting them in a heat-proof bowl, pouring boiling water over, counting slowly to 30 then draining them - works every time, the skins slip off easily as long as the tomatoes are ripe.

Remove the core and seeds from the tomatoes, discard and chop the flesh roughly.

Place the chorizo in a medium-sized, non-stick oven-proof sauté pan and cook over a low heat, turning regularly until the slices release their oils. Lift the chorizo out with a slotted spoon, wrap in a few sheets of kitchen paper to mop up the excess oil and set aside.

Add the butter to the pan and once melted add the onions and peppers and cook over a low heat until soft.

Add the mushrooms, turn the heat up and stir briskly until the mushrooms, onions and pepper are slightly caramelised around the edges.

Turn the heat back to low, add the tomato and chorizo, mix well and allow everything to continue at a very low simmer.

Lightly beat the eggs in a bowl, add a good pinch of salt and a few grindings of black pepper, mix well and pour into the pan.

Make sure the egg covers everything (push the other ingredients down into the liquid) then transfer to the middle of the oven and bake, uncovered for 5 minutes.

Remove the pan from the oven, turn on the grill, scatter the cheese on top of the omelette, place the pan on a low shelf, keep an eye on it and when the cheese is nicely browned and bubbling turn the heat off.

Transfer to a warmed serving plate (a fish slice or spatula helps here!)

~

Some can sling a classic omelette together in a matter of minutes, others simply refuse to go there! Baking an omelette is the answer for those of us who feel a bit challenged (and I include myself here!) Feel free to sling in whatever is in the fridge, freezer or cupboard plus it makes a great early morning meal the next day - just thinly slice what is left from the night before and pop them into the oven for 5 minutes or so...

Salmon Kedgeree

(makes 2 servings)

INGREDIENTS

- 2 x Omega 3-rich eggs
- 375ml fish or vegetable stock
- 1 salmon steak or fillet (skin on)
- I small onion, peeled and finely sliced
- 2 dill fronds
- 1 inch/2.5cm piece fresh ginger, peeled and grated
- Juice of half a lemon
- 1 tablespoon avocado oil
- 6 spring onions, cleaned and finely sliced
- ¼ teaspoon ground cumin
- ¼ teaspoon ground coriander
- ¼ teaspoon ground turmeric
- 200g white basmati rice
- 2 handfuls baby spinach leaves
- 2 handfuls flaked almonds

METHOD

Place the eggs in a pot of cold water, bring slowly to the boil, turn the heat down to a gentle bubble and cook for 5 minutes then run the pot under cold water until the eggs cool slightly, drain and set aside.

Pour the stock into a shallow sauté pan, add the onion, dill, ginger, lemon juice, a pinch of sea salt and a few good grindings of black pepper and bring slowly to the boil.

Turn the heat to a gentle simmer, place the salmon on top (skin side down), cover the pan with a lid or foil and cook for 10-15 minutes or until the salmon is cooked to your liking.

Meanwhile, warm the avocado oil in another sauté pan over a medium heat, add the spring onions, the spices and a pinch of sea salt and cook, stirring regularly until the spring onions are soft.

Add the rice and stir well before turning the heat to very low and continuing to simmer very gently.

When the salmon is cooked, lift it out onto a plate, remove the skin and cover with foil to keep it warm.

Strain the liquid into the rice and spice mixture, turn up the heat a little and simmer for 15 minutes or until the rice is cooked but still has a slight bite to it.

Quickly toast the flaked almonds in a dry frying pan over a gentle heat until golden and crunchy before turning off the heat.

Flake the salmon and add to the rice along with the spinach, stir gently and simmer for another 5 minutes or until the fish is well-warmed through and the spinach has wilted.

Quickly peel the boiled eggs and chop them roughly before adding to the kedgeree.

~

If you like kedgeree, you'll love this! It's pretty filling and super-rich in healthy fats. If it's a 'hungry night', add a bit more salmon (tinned is fine), stir in a spoonful of natural yoghurt to make the whole thing a little more 'fluid' and sling a few more nuts on top to add a bit more crunch and a few more healthy fats.

Soft Boiled Eggs with Sweet Potato and Avocado

(makes 2 servings)

INGREDIENTS

- ½ large sweet potato, peeled and cut into 4 lengthwise slices
- Sea salt and freshly ground black pepper
- 2 large omega 3-rich or organic, free range eggs
- ½ large or 1 small ripe avocado, stoned and flesh scooped from skin

- ½ tablespoon fresh lime juice
- ½ tablespoon coriander leaves, finely chopped

METHOD

Preheat the oven to 200C/400F/Gas Mark 6.

Paint both sides of the sweet potato slices with oil, sprinkle with salt and pepper and bake (turning regularly) until nice and crispy on both sides but still soft in the middle (around 15 minutes).

Meanwhile, boil your eggs.

My method: Prick the eggs on the rounded bottom, place in a small pan, cover with cold water, bring slowly to the boil and the minute the water starts to boil, turn the heat down so that it is just bubbling gently and set the timer for 3 minutes. As soon as the timer goes off, remove from the heat, drain and run lots of cold water over the eggs, before draining and setting aside. Works every time!

If you want them a little less runny, go for 4 minutes, hard-boiled, go for 5. Also... an egg piercer is a brilliant and very cheap investment that lasts pretty much forever!

Mash the avocado in a bowl with a fork, add the lime juice and coriander and mash some more until it has a chunky but silky texture.

Shell and half the eggs, place 2 slices of sweet potato on each plate, top with a good scoop of the avocado mix then place 2 egg halves on top and another pinch of salt and a few twists of black pepper.

A fresh tomato and basil salad simply dressed with extra virgin olive oil, a splash of lemon juice and some salt and pepper goes really well with this.

~

This may seem like quite an unusual mix but trust me, it tastes really good!

Mid Morning and Mid Afternoon Snacks

- a small pot of hummus with a selection of raw vegetable sticks
- a small bowl of mixed olives with feta cheese cubes
- a glass of fresh tomato juice with a handful of fresh, mixed nuts
- a cold boiled egg
- 1 celery stick filled with nut butter
- 2 oatcakes or rice cakes topped with nut butter, mashed avocado or tzatziki and smoked salmon
- a small carton of natural yoghurt with 2 tablespoons of berries or mixed chopped fresh fruit and a scattering of fresh nuts
- 2 thick discs of cucumber, tomato, radish, courgette or apple topped with hummus, nut butter or soft goats cheese
- a small carton of natural cottage cheese mixed with diced fresh pear and crushed walnuts
- 2 protein/energy balls - make sure they have no added sugars
- half a small, ripe avocado filled with tinned tuna mixed with natural yoghurt
- 2 nut-stuffed dates
- a mug of miso soup
- 2 slices of hard cheese with a handful of green grapes
- 2 handfuls of sprouted grains or beans

Bedtime and Bedside Snacks

- 2 oatcakes with 2 thin slices of cold, cooked turkey
- a small carton of natural yoghurt with one teaspoon runny honey
- half a banana on its own or mashed onto one rice cake

- a handful of fresh cherries and/or a glass of Morello cherry juice
- 1 egg scrambled on 1 rye cracker
- a small bowl of creamy porridge
- a small glass of **essential smoothie**

Drinks

Hot Lemon and Ginger

Boil the kettle, put 1 or 2 tablespoons of freshly-squeezed lemon or lime juice in a mug (the stuff that comes in bottles or squeezy lemon/lime shapes is fine), add a good pinch of sea salt crystals, grate in some peeled fresh root ginger (you can peel it, cut it into chunks, bag these and freeze, then grate from frozen), add boiling water, stir well, leave to cool a little before stirring in a teaspoon of Manuka honey and sipping slowly.

Cleansing Juice

Mix equal quantities of water, unsweetened grapefruit, pomegranate and cranberry juices in a large glass. Add a pinch of cinnamon, ginger and allspice and stir well. You can also warm it through gently and have it as a hot drink on a cold day.

Switchel

Mix 2 tablespoons apple cider vinegar, 3 tablespoons maple syrup, the juice of half a lime and a 5cm piece of fresh ginger, peeled and grated in a large mug. Top up with boiling water, stir well, cover and refrigerate overnight. Serve over ice and top up with sparkling water.

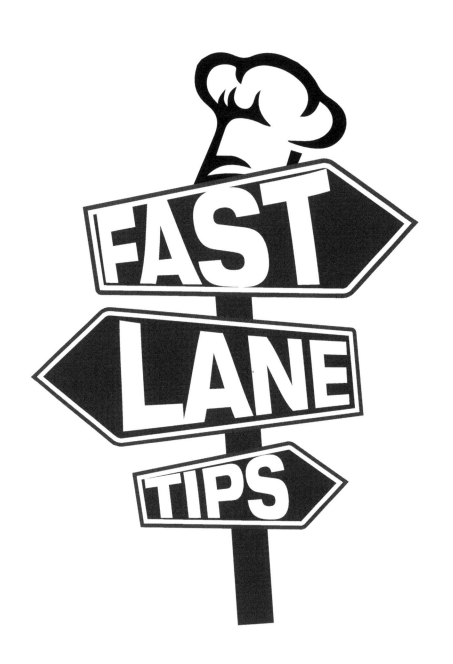

Soup Makes an Impressive Difference!

A soup a day is a brilliant way to get more vegetables into your day!

Keep repeating this phrase until it becomes indelibly fixed in your brain!

The creation of nearly all soups start with sautéing at least 2 vegetables for the soup base - onions, celery, leeks, carrots, garlic etc. Then there is the addition of another 2 or 3 or more either during the cooking or towards the end, so already you are looking at quite a few portions of vegetables!

All the soup recommendations in your diet plan plus those suggested for 'keeping the diet going' are vegetable-rich so simply by having a bowl-a-day and perhaps adding a cup or a mug as a snack, you can fret a little less about getting your recommended daily quota.

ARE YOU A SOUP-MAKING VIRGIN?

I come across people on a regular basis who tell me that they don't or can't make soup which, because I have been making soups since I was a teen and you are unlikely to ever find my fridge or freezer without one or two bowls or bags lurking in there somewhere, I find difficult to get my head around but then again, I relish spending an hour of my free time creating a couple of delicious and nutritious soups whilst catching up on my recorded TV favourites - different strokes as they say!

Soup-making is ridiculously simple and straightforward - little can go wrong - so start with my *pea, mint and lettuce* or *spinach and watercress* or *light chicken or lentil broth* and your confidence will soar!

Don't Get Caught in the Empty Fridge Trap!

Some people are extremely organised and rarely seem to find themselves in that place where there's nothing other than a tired-looking lettuce and a few past their sell by date packets of cold meat in the fridge and a bag of peas in the freezer! Others (and I include myself here) are not always quite as on the ball as we might be!

Studies show that even when we are only at home (and awake) for a mere 5 hours in every 24, we open the fridge door somewhere between 10 and 20 times, looking for some sort of sustenance - so an empty fridge is never going to work if fat loss is the goal - we simply head for the cereals, crisps or biscuits!

I like a shopping app - what a marvellous invention! You use the last few grains of rice or the last tin of chopped tomatoes and all you have to do is enter it into the app on your tablet or phone and it's all there tomorrow just waiting for you to become that fabulously-organised person you always knew was in there somewhere! And... better still, you can share many of these apps with others in your household so it's just a matter of a quick text to say "sorry, working late, leave you to pick up dinner?" Genius!

How to Throw Fat Busting Meals Together in Record Time!

The number one priority has to be a bit of planning. Not always easy but it makes such a difference!

If you enjoy cooking and you cook on a regular basis, it's likely you keep a good stock of the essentials in the cupboard and in the freezer and this is a vital piece of the jigsaw when you are on a mission to lose weight.

I recommend you work on a week to week basis, plan your meals and snacks, take 10 minutes to check your stores and keep a note of everything that needs replenishing on your shopping app or in your notes/reminders on your phone and simply do one reasonably 'big shop' for the week. That leaves you in a place where it's only the fresh foods that need to be picked up every couple of days.

If you have a big kitchen with big cupboards and a big freezer - lucky you - you can buy stuff in bulk and save money! But even if you are short of space, with a little careful planning you can ensure that every inch of it holds everything you need and nothing you don't need.

Most of my recipes plus my meal and snack recommendations focus on easy-to-find ingredients. There are a few which require a little more *dedicated shopping time* but generally-speaking, you can substitute, so if there is a dish that includes foods you are unfamiliar with or know are going to be hard to find, don't panic - just try a few alternatives and all should be fine.

Many of us don't really make best use of the freezer but no matter how small, it is a godsend!

Keep a stock of freezer bags (large, medium and small) and **plastic boxes with lids** (inexpensive, reusable and stack nicely for clever space-saving) - and make sure you have a **marker pen** so you know what's in the bags and boxes! Also extremely useful and inexpensive are a stock of **ice cube trays**.

Frozen vegetables are tops for quick meals and there are a vast selection of ready-bagged varieties available but you can freeze just about any variety bought fresh from the market or supermarket or if any that are lurking in the fridge/vegetable rack are beginning to look a little tired. **Top Tip**: chop them into chunks and bag them in one layer then freeze flat - once frozen they can be stacked taking up minimal space.

Frozen fruits also come ready-bagged and are great for smoothies, compotes and fruity sauces and as with fresh vegetables, you can chop or slice most fresh varieties - particularly those that may be making the fruit bowl look a little sad - freeze them flat and stack them.

Most dairy products freeze well when fresh (not yoghurt) and as I recommend you include these in your diet on a regular basis but not in large amounts, the freezer really is your friend here as you can small-bag, small-box or small-bottle them (those little plastic bottles used for shop-bought smoothies are great - just wash them thoroughly in plenty of hot water and reuse for milks and creams). Similarly, keep your cheese consumption under control by cubing or grating your favourites and storing in portions.

Lots of great things can be frozen in ice cube trays before being bagged - and - most can be added during the cooking process whilst still frozen: chopped fresh herbs (fill half of each cube and top up with extra virgin olive oil), pestos, marinades and the remainder of any sauces you make. This is a particularly helpful little trick when you discover dishes that you particularly enjoy and want to repeat.

Cooked grains, beans and lentils are also great freezer standbys. Again, freezing them flat in a bag allows for easy stacking and lots of space-saving.

I am not a big fan of freezing my recipes or recommended meals in their entirety - most of them are best freshly made - **but my soups, casseroles and curries are an exception** (they are born to be frozen in portions for convenience and reusable soup bags are invaluable, particularly if you are transporting them for reheating later in the day!)

Plus... I swear by a quickly-defrosted mug of good, nourishing miso broth (make it in bulk using sachets or pastes and freeze in cup or mug-sized portions) to take the edge off any gut-wrenching hunger or uncontrollable snack attacks that often occur around early evening before you start to get dinner ready!

Obviously, I recommend you stick as closely as possible to your diet plan for the first 2 weeks and that means you are best advised to have everything you need in stock but **you don't have to be a slave to the process.** If you suddenly discover you don't have something in stock, either miss it out or substitute with something similar or be a little inventive with whatever is in the fridge, freezer and/or cupboard!

Top Tip: when all else fails, a great and very quick and nourishing meal can be thrown together with tinned beans, lentils or chickpeas, tinned tomatoes, quick-cook brown rice, 'very lazy' garlic, ginger and chillies (which keep in the fridge for ages), frozen mixed vegetables and a scattering of whatever nuts and seeds you have about.

BOWL IT, BOX IT, BAG IT OR PLATE IT?

Bowls appear to have taken over the planet as the **vessel of choice** for a health-enhancing and fat busting breakfast, lunch, dinner or quick snack and it's not difficult to understand why!

Any reader who is familiar with my recipes will be only-too-aware that bowls of food (particularly soups, stews and salads) have always played a major part in my diets and there are good reasons behind this...

Firstly: soup is a messy affair in anything other than a bowl (although I am also a fan of a mug or cup or soup flask!)

Secondly: food looks good in a bowl and you don't have to be a whizz on the 'plating-up' front to create something that looks appealing.

Thirdly: you can **build a dish** very successfully in a bowl. Either **start with a base** of leaves or vegetables or grains, **add a middle** of protein, play around with all manner of **toppings** - and - if there is a sauce or a dressing, a bowl ensures this stays in place rather than running uncontrollably around a plate!

Alternatively, you can **position your food** within the bowl so that everything has its own private corner which also makes your meal come alive!

Lastly: it's quick, easy, generally doesn't require more than one piece of cutlery and leaves your other hand free when you are eating. Of course, **taking your time over a meal and not trying to multitask** will always be the best route to good digestion and maximum nourishment **but** time is not always on our side!

BOXING AND BAGGING ALSO GET MY VOTE!

As long as you have a few decent-sized food containers with secure lids, you can transport your meals and snacks to work or when you know you have to be out for a good chunk of the day (always best to have a few in the cupboard as it is all too easy to leave one at the office, on the train or in the car!)

Now... you may be one of those types who want to emulate some of those oh-so-organised and beautiful-looking lunch boxes which are compartmentalised and look quite superb on Instagram and Pinterest and if so - crack on! I myself, am much more of a throw it all into a box before you head to bed and let all the ingredients feel the love for each other overnight in the fridge type of luncher or snacker - I am not overly bothered about someone passing by and commenting that my lunch looks like a bit of a 'dog's dinner' in their view - as long as it tastes good and keeps me going through the afternoon, I'm happy!

But this is important... most sauces and dressings should be kept separate (and yes you'll need another little container with a good and secure lid or a small jam jar for these!) before being added and mixed through just before you dive into your box of healthy and energising goodness.

Small soup bags are superb and not just for soups! Good quality soup bags are not just sturdy, dependable and don't leak, they are also reusable which makes them a fabulously-inexpensive investment. You can simply give them a good wash with detergent, a serious rinsing with hot water and they are ready for the next batch of soups, stews or casseroles you want to freeze or refrigerate in portions or to fill with a nice wee tasty salad or snack to pop in your handbag or briefcase. I use *Lakeland Soup'n'Sauce* bags **www.lakeland.co.uk** which have never let me down but there are plenty more great products out there - a quick internet search will head you in the right direction.

A Few More Words About Sugar!

It's not a weight loss friend, in fact it's not really much of a friend at all! But it's kind of nice and it's kind of hard to say no to! And it's not really our fault that we like it - we are hard-wired to like it! Often, the only way our hunter/gatherer ancestors were able to tell whether a fruit or berry from a bush or tree was poisonous or not was to have a tiny taste and generally-speaking, if it was sweet it was likely just fine. Then... there's breast milk which is wonderfully-sweet so those of us who were breast-fed learned to love a bit of sweetness very early on.

However, things have gone a bit awry and sugar is everywhere and is now added to everything from fizzy drinks to breads to cereals to sauces to soups and even fries which unfortunately means that not only is it hard to spot but also puts us in that difficult place where our sugar receptors have gone into overdrive - and are loving every sweet moment!

Some suggest that sugar is like a drug and there's something in that. The more we have, the more we want and the harder we try to wean ourselves off it, the harder it can be to deal with cravings.

What's important to remember is that the brain loves sugar - it's a glutton for any foods that are either rich in natural sugars or those that have added sugars.

So what can we do in a bid to satisfy a desire for something sweet occasionally without encouraging the brain to think that every day is a sugar-fest?

I suppose the best answer is that **every learned habit can become**

an unlearned habit thanks to the massive capabilities of the human brain - but it can take a little time and going cold turkey can have disastrous consequences!

I am going to suggest that if you have been a bit of a sugar-head for some considerable time, you often struggle with energy dips, blood sugar spikes, cravings and can't think straight unless you eat something sweet.

Like it or not, you are likely to find cutting added sugars out of your life relatively hard and **going cold turkey may not be the route for you.** Think headaches, mind-numbing fatigue and low mood and you might be close - so - here's what I recommend in the early stages...

Follow your diet plan as closely as you can each day and when the desire for something sweet threatens to overtake, have one of the following:

- a piece of very sweet, fresh fruit (mango, peach, nectarine, papaya, pawpaw, grapes, banana, pineapple, kiwi, strawberries, lychees) with a handful of fresh sweet nuts
- an oatcake or rye cracker with no added sugar peanut or almond butter
- a small pot of natural Greek yoghurt with a generous swirl of runny honey
- a mini bar of very dark chocolate and a handful of mixed seeds
- a couple of nut-stuffed dates
- a fruit and yoghurt smoothie
- a small slice of good quality, freshly-baked carrot cake or banana bread (no icing)

Each of the above offer something that will quickly satisfy a yearning for something sweet but are also combined with some protein and/or fat so you don't experience a major blood sugar spike and most require little or no preparation.

You might be surprised at just how quickly your sweet tooth starts to become less invasive and once it does, things really do get a lot easier!

Indulge and Enjoy!

Imagining a life without the occasional treat doesn't work long term. It can be relatively easy short term when you are really determined but let's not pretend that you can give up treats forever and become saint-like (there are some who can but I have a tiny suspicion they are not reading this book!)

A brilliant route to take here is when you know a bit of indulgence is likely on the cards (holidays, special events, social occasions etc), you make every bite and sip count. Indulgence is all about enjoyment so when you do it, you have to relish it before moving back to your slightly more controlled diet life!

Don't fall into the trap of eating or drinking something that merely ticks the 'averagely-good' box just because it's right in front of you - go for the very best you can afford or find and rather than chastising yourself for having indulged, really savour the moment then move on - it's a treat but it doesn't happen every day!

Don't let the Diet Saboteurs Grind You Down!

There are always going to be people out there who are right by your side when you are working your butt and mind off to get fitter, feel better and lose weight - but - there are also always going to be those that don't relish your progress and try to make things difficult with phrases like "surely one doughnut won't hurt" - this is when you have to stay strong!

Make your food decisions fast and stick to them and feel free to contact me if you are struggling - I can't guarantee that I will get back to you right at that 'difficult moment' but I will get back to you and lend a helping hand or give you a few relatively convincing excuses to throw into the conversation and get you out of trouble!

How to Keep the Diet Going After 2 Weeks

Your 14 days are now up but you still have some weight/fat to lose so what happens next?

You have likely found a few favourite meals and snacks and worked out which ones fit in with your days. You will also have determined how much time you have for shopping, prepping and cooking and (with luck) determined when you can steal a little time to do a bit of forward planning in a bid to be ahead of the game and 'bag' a few of your chosen meals and snacks so you are rarely facing an empty fridge, freezer or cupboard.

You may also have had to factor in a couple of **Grab and Go Days** and if so, I hope my recommended snacks did the trick - it's a good idea is to keep a list of them to hand or on your smartphone to steer you in the right direction!

You may also have had a few **Soup and Juice Days with a 14 hour 'no eating' window** which okay I admit, require a little bit of planning but I bet you felt good and just a little bit smug at the end of the day! They are a great little tactic to have up your sleeve when things go a bit pear-shaped or there has perhaps been a little too much indulgence!

THERE ARE LOTS OF THINGS YOU CAN DO STARTING RIGHT NOW!

- you can start all over again and repeat days 1 to 14

- you can make a list of the meals and snacks that you like and stick with them

- you can throw in a few **Soup and Juice Days** in a row as long as you know your timetable isn't going to be too hectic

- you can throw in a few **Grab and Go Days** in a row if time is really tight and you just know that prepping and cooking is not likely to happen

- you can keep referring back to the 20 'changes' I recommend and continue to factor in as many as you can

- you can go to my website **www.fionakirk.com** where you will find more fat-busting recipes if you want to mix things up a bit

- you can contact me through my website or social media pages if you are unsure of any of my recommendations or want me to suggest any alterations to my recipes to suit your tastes

Just keep in mind that it is the combination of changes you make to your diet and lifestyle over as short a period of time as possible - and the continuation of them - that result in improved health and successful weight loss, fat loss and inches off hips, bums and bellies!

A QUICK REMINDER!

Come On! 3 More Vegetables Per Day!

Don't Forget Fruit

Go To Work on an Egg

Go Nuts for Calcium and Magnesium

Play Clever With Starch

Drink Water Before Meals and Snacks

Step Away from the Fizzy Stuff!

Lunch on Lentils and Beans

Pack in the Protein

Feel Fuller Faster with Fats

Love Your Curries!

Make Coffee Count

Think Pink!

More Sleep = Faster Fat Loss

Make Exercise Count

Have a Soup and Juice Day

The Hot Topic of Vitamin D

Change Your Cooking Methods

The Alcohol Debate

To Supplement or Not to Supplement?

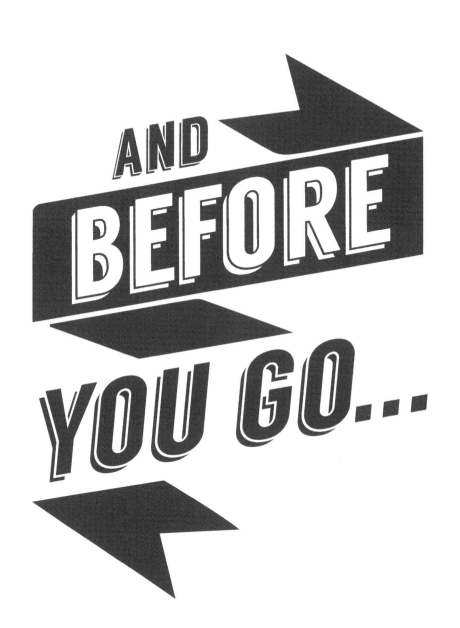

AND BEFORE YOU GO...

Big Thanks to My Amazing Team of Worker Bees!

For fabulous food photography and the ability to create my videos despite me continually forgetting my script and invariably falling about laughing! *Keny Drew* **eastneukglass.com**

For the design of all my book covers and endless hours of book design and often working into the wee small hours of the night on the other side of the world when the publication deadline is upon us! *Max Morris* **milkbar-creative.com**

For all my PR and publicity and for his extraordinary patience, exhaustive support and great friendship over the last 11 years. *David Clarke* **rock-pr.com**

For taking care of all my social media and my blog plus that rare skill of making the client believe that they are not 'lost in the dark ages' on the social media front! *Gemma Kirk*

For spending who knows how many hours turning my many books into who knows how many formats for sale through eBook retailers! *Alan Cooper* **yourebookpartners.com**

My Books, Blog and Social Media Links

MY BOOKS

(see **www.fionakirk.com** *and click on BOOKS to find out more!)*

The New 2 Weeks in the Fast Lane Diet
Eat Live & Lose the Flab
Soup Can Make You Thin: The Diet
Soup Can Make You Thin: The Cookbook
2 Weeks in the Super Fast Lane
Fast and Fabulous Fat Loss
Diet Secrets Uncovered for Seniors

Diet Secrets Uncovered for Menopausal Women
Diet Secrets Uncovered for Office Workers
Diet Secrets Uncovered for Single Men and Women
Diet Secrets Uncovered for Newly Weds
Diet Secrets Uncovered for Women Post Pregnancy
Diet Secrets Uncovered for Stressed Executives
Diet Secrets Uncovered for Fitness Enthusiasts
Diet Secrets Uncovered for Shift Workers
Diet Secrets Uncovered for Teenagers

MY BLOG

*(see **www.fionakirk.com** and click on BLOG to keep up to date with diet news and to subscribe to my free monthly newsletters!)*

MY SOCIAL MEDIA LINKS

FACEBOOK: **/fionakirkbooks**
TWITTER: **@fatbustforever**
INSTAGRAM: **@fionamkirk**
LINKEDIN: **/fionakirknutritionist**

Quiz Answers

1. **c**	6. **b**	11. **c**	16. **c**
2. **b**	7. **b**	12. **c**	17. **a**
3. **b**	8. **d**	13. **a**	18. **b**
4. **c**	9. **d**	14. **b**	19. **c**
5. **c**	10. **b**	15. **b**	20. **b**

Most Common Signs of Possible Vitamin and Mineral Deficiency

Vitamin A

mouth ulcers

poor night vision

acne

frequent colds and infections

dry flaky skin

dandruff

thrush or cystitis

diarrhoea

Vitamin B1

tender muscles

eye pains

prickly legs

stomach pains

constipation

tingling hands

rapid heartbeat

Vitamin B2

burning or gritty eyes

sensitivity to bright lights

sore tongue

dull or oily hair

eczema or dermatitis

split nails

cracked lips

Vitamin B3

lack of energy

diarrhoea

insomnia

headaches or migraines

bleeding or tender gums

acne

eczema or dermatitis

Vitamin B5

muscle tremors or cramps

burning feet or tender heels

nausea or vomiting

exhaustion after light exercise

teeth-grinding

Vitamin B6

infrequent dream recall

water retention

tingling hands

muscle tremors or cramps

lack of energy

flaky skin

Vitamin B12

poor hair condition
eczema or dermatitis
mouth oversensitive to heat or cold
lack of energy
constipation
tender or sore muscles
pale skin

Folic Acid

anaemia
eczema
cracked lips
prematurely greying hair
lack of energy
poor appetite
stomach pains

Biotin

dry skin
poor hair condition
prematurely greying hair
tender of sore muscles
poor appetite or nausea
eczema or dermatitis

Vitamin C

frequent colds and/or infections
lack of energy
bleeding or tender gums
easy bruising
nosebleeds
slow wound-healing
red pimples on skin

Vitamin D

joint pain or stiffness
backache
tooth decay
muscle cramps
hair loss

Vitamin E

lack of sex drive
exhaustion after light exercise
easy bruising
slow wound-healing
varicose veins
loss of muscle tone
infertility

Vitamin K

easy bleeding
easy bruising

Calcium

muscle tremors or cramps
insomnia
joint pain or arthritis
tooth decay
high blood pressure

Chromium

excessive hot and/or cold sweats
dizziness or irritability after a few hours without food
cold hands
drowsiness during the day
excessive thirst
addiction to sweet foods

Iron

pale skin
sore tongue
fatigue
listlessness
loss of appetite
nausea
sensitivity to cold

Magnesium

muscle tremors or spasms
muscle weakness
insomnia
high blood pressure
irregular heartbeat
constipation
hyperactivity

Manganese

muscle twitches
dizziness or poor sense of balance
sore knees
joint pain

Potassium

irregular heartbeat
muscle weakness
pins and needles
nausea
diarrhoea
swollen abdomen

Selenium

family history of cancer
signs of premature ageing
cataracts
high blood pressure
frequent infections

Sodium

dizziness
heat exhaustion
low blood pressure
rapid pulse
muscle cramps
nausea
headaches

Zinc

poor sense of taste or smell
white marks on fingernails
frequent infections
stretch marks
acne or greasy skin
loss of appetite
tendency to depression

Omega Fats

dry skin
eczema
dry hair or dandruff
excessive thirst
PMS or breast pain
water retention

Co-enzyme Q10

lack of energy

poor immune health

poor exercise tolerance

family history of heart disease

Printed in Great Britain
by Amazon